SK277 Human Biology
Science: Level 2

The Open University

This publication forms part of an Open University course SK277 *Human biology*. The complete list of texts which make up this course can be found at the back. Details of this and other Open University courses can be obtained from the Student Registration and Enquiry Service, The Open University, PO Box 197, Milton Keynes MK7 6BJ, United Kingdom: tel. +44 (0)870 333 4340, email general-enquiries@open.ac.uk

Alternatively, you may visit the Open University website at http://www.open.ac.uk where you can learn more about the wide range of courses and packs offered at all levels by The Open University.

To purchase a selection of Open University course materials visit www.ouw.co.uk, or contact Open University Worldwide, Walton Hall, Milton Keynes MK7 6AA, United Kingdom for a brochure (tel. +44 (0)1908 858793; fax +44 (0)1908 858787; email ouw-customer-services@open.ac.uk).

The Open University
Walton Hall, Milton Keynes
MK7 6AA

First published 2004. Second edition 2006.

Edited and designed by The Open University.

Typeset by The Open University.

Printed in the United Kingdom by Latimer Trend and Company Ltd, Plymouth.

The paper used in this publication is procured from forests independently certified to the level of Forest Stewardship Council (FSC) principles and criteria. Chain of custody certification allows the tracing of this paper back to specific forest-management units (see www.fsc.org).

ISBN 978 0 7492 1879 9

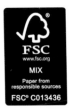

3.2

THE COURSE TEAM

Course Team Chair and Academic Editor

Heather McLannahan

Course Managers

Alastair Ewing

Colin Walker

Course Team Assistants

Catherine Eden

Rebecca Efthimiou

Course Team Authors

Patricia Ash

Pete Clifton

Paul Gabbott

Nicolette Habgood

Tim Halliday

Heather McLannahan

Kerry Murphy

Daniel Nettle

Payam Rezaie

Other Contributors

Vickie Arrowsmith

Leslie Baillie

Production and Presentation Manager

John Owen

Project Manager

Judith Pickering

Editors

Rebecca Graham

Gillian Riley

Bina Sharma

Margaret Swithenby

Design

Sarah Hofton

Jenny Nockles

Illustration

Steve Best

Pam Owen

CD-ROM Production

Phil Butcher

Will Rawes

External Course Assessor

Dinah Gould

Picture Researcher

Lydia Eaton

Indexer

Jane Henley

Course Website

Patrina Law

Louise Olney

SK277 *Human Biology* makes use of material originally produced for SK220 *Human Biology and Health* by the following individuals: Janet Bunker, Melanie Clements, Basiro Davey, Brian Goodwin, Linda Jones, Jeanne Katz, Heather McLannahan, Hilary MacQueen, Jill Saffrey, Moyra Sidell, Michael Stewart, Margaret Swithenby and Frederick Toates.

CONTENTS

CHAPTER I

DIVERSITY AND CHANGE

Learning Outcomes

After completing this chapter, you should be able to:

1.1 Describe the sources of variability between individuals.

1.2 Explain how mutation, independent assortment and recombination can promote genetic variation in human populations.

1.3 Describe how point and frame shift genetic mutations arise.

1.4 Outline how chromosome abnormalities may arise during meiosis.

1.5 Explain how genetic and environmental variables may interact to produce variability both within and across generations.

1.6 Apply an understanding of gene–environment interactions to possible explanations of variability in human body weight and adiposity, ageing and to other areas covered in the course.

1.1 Introduction

Humans, like other organisms, are variable (Figure 1.1). The variation extends from physical characteristics such as height, weight or skin colour, to physiological measures such as cholesterol level, liability to diseases such as breast cancer, response to drug treatments, and even to the complex characteristics that make up our personality. In addition, each of us changes over our lifetime, both physically and mentally. In each case we know that environmental variables interact with individual genetic differences to produce long-lasting differences between individual members of our species. The complete set of characteristics of an organism is described as its **phenotype.** The idea that at least some of the variability between individuals is genetic and heritable and leads to differences in biological fitness lies at the core of Darwin's theory of evolution by natural selection.

In Book 1 (Section 2.9.3), we examined the way in which cells within the body multiply through mitosis. A key point about this process is that it generates two new cells that are genetically identical to the original cell through the process of DNA replication. Moreover, the new cells also tend to inherit the particular patterns of gene activation from the original cell. In this way, liver cells within a particular individual can divide to give further liver cells whereas gut epithelial cells divide to give further gut epithelial cells, despite the fact that both types of cell share the identical set of genes. Of course, these new cells may change their appearance and function as they continue to differentiate or age, and this will also be reflected in different patterns of gene activation, but the genes themselves will normally remain unchanged.

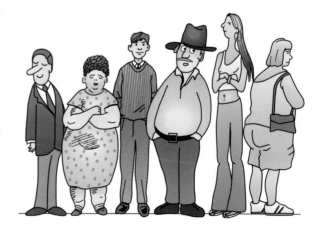

Figure 1.1 Diversity of shape and size in humans.

So how does genetic variation arise? This is the topic of the first section of this chapter. You have already met the role that mutations, which are changes in DNA structure, can have in the origin of cancer. The accumulation of a few such changes, perhaps in the cells of the breast or pancreas, can lead to the uncontrolled growth characteristic of a cancer (Book 1, Section 2.13). Although such mutations cannot outlive the individual in which they occur, mutations that occur in the **germ cells** (the gametes and their precursor cells) can be passed on to succeeding generations. These mutations in the germ cells, though more often harmful, may sometimes be beneficial. In either case, they provide the inherited variability that is essential for the process of natural selection.

The process of cell division that gives rise to the gametes is quite different to that which gives rise to new **somatic** cells (i.e. cells of the body). It is known as **meiosis** and generates cells containing just a single copy of each chromosome rather than the pairs that are found in somatic cells (as shown in Figure 2.12 of Book 1). In Section 1.2.2 of this chapter we shall see that an important aspect of meiosis is that it allows alleles to be exchanged between the two members of these chromosomal pairs – thus generating new combinations of alleles on the individual chromosomes that are later incorporated into the gametes. This is a random process that is called **recombination**. In addition, the chromosomes assort independently during meiosis resulting in some of the chromosomes within the gamete deriving from the mother of the individual who is producing the gametes and others from the father of this individual. This **independent assortment** is another random process, very similar to shuffling a pack of playing cards and then dealing them out to the card players. The selection of cards that each player receives will contain some black cards and some red cards, each card being unique and having a different value. The cards in a selection are independent of each other; for example, you do not necessarily receive an equal number of each colour of card, and if you were to look at just one of the cards in a selection it would not enable you to know about any other card in that same selection. In other words, the cards have assorted independently of one another. These processes of recombination of alleles within a chromosome and independent assortment of chromosomes produce additional variation that is thought to be one of the critical long-term evolutionary advantages of sexual over asexual reproduction. However, it is also true that particularly advantageous combinations of alleles, especially when they are on different chromosomes, may be lost due to recombination and independent assortment during meiosis in succeeding generations.

● Why might genetic variability be of long-term advantage to a species?

● Environments change – if variation exists within a population then maybe some individuals will survive in the new situation. The idea that at least some of the variability between individuals is genetic and heritable and leads to differences in biological fitness in different environments lies at the heart of the theory of evolution by natural selection (see Book 1, Section 1.4.2).

In a natural environment, which is subject to climatic forces that can cause occasional shortages of food or lead to unexpected extremes of temperature, individuals with unusual combinations of alleles may be especially well adapted and likely to survive such hard times, when most of the population dies. There is genetic evidence that our own species went through such a population bottleneck and nearly became extinct around 70 000–100 000 years ago.

Section 1.3 of this chapter will consider how these central ideas in modern biology might illuminate our understanding of individual differences in body weight. We will look at examples of the way in which either genetic or environmental variation may make obesity more likely, and then briefly consider the implications of this knowledge for the treatment of obesity. Section 1.4 of the chapter will shift the focus from 'diversity' to 'change', with an emphasis on the gradual alterations of function that occur as humans age. But first we need to understand more about the sources of variability that lead to the production of the unique gametes.

1.2 Sources of variation

In this section we will look at the origins of genetic diversity between individuals and also the way in which this genetic diversity interacts with environmental variables to produce the range of variation found in any particular character.

1.2.1 Mutation

Mutations, which are changes in the structure of the DNA making up a single gene or group of genes, are the ultimate source of all genetic variability. Almost all of a cell's DNA is found within the chromosomes in the nucleus of the cell. A chromosome consists of the two paired strands of DNA that are organized as a double helix (Book 1, Section 2.6). However, a small amount of DNA is also found in the mitochondria of the cell (see Section 4.3.3 for more details). The individual nucleotides that make up a strand of DNA use a triplet code (the *codon*) to represent the ordering of the 20 or so amino acids from which proteins are constructed. The codon has 64 possible combinations, and most of the amino acids can be generated by more than one combination – this is often described as a 'redundant' code. From this you can imagine that a mistake in copying a single base (nucleotide) when DNA replicates would change the code at that point. Such changes are known as **point mutations** (compare Figure 1.2a and b). Sometimes they will have no effect because the changed triplet will still code for the original amino acid. In other cases the protein will have a single different amino acid that may substantially alter its properties.

The first example of a point mutation to be clearly understood in these terms was a change in one of the globin proteins that make up haemoglobin. The mutation causes **sickle cell anaemia** and also provides some degree of protection from infection by the mosquito-borne parasite that causes malaria. This mutation is widely distributed in areas where malaria is endemic. Individuals who have two copies of the mutated gene suffer from severe anaemia (see Case Report 1.1), whereas individuals with only one mutated and one normal gene (i.e. having two different alleles) have a milder anaemia together with partial protection from malaria infection. This means that their overall biological fitness is higher than that of individuals with two normal genes, who are more likely to contract and die from malaria, and also of individuals with two mutated genes, who may die as a result of their anaemia. This is why the mutation has been favoured by natural selection and remains within the populations in areas in which malaria is endemic.

Haemoglobin is made up of two pairs of polypeptide chains (alpha and beta) as shown in Figure 3.5 of Book 3. The beta chain is 146 amino acids long, and the change that produces sickling is in the 6th amino acid which is changed from glutamic acid to valine. This change results from a single point substitution of the adenine for thymine at the appropriate position in the gene for beta globin on chromosome 11. There are many other examples of mutations due to substitution of one base with another arising from point mutations and we shall examine an example relevant to obesity later in the chapter.

Point mutations are not the only type of change that can occur in the DNA sequences that make a gene. Another possible error that can occur is that one nucleotide will be missed out during the copying process in meiosis or mitosis (Figure 1.2c). The effects of this type of mutation are likely to be very much more serious than a point mutation.

● Why is the loss of a nucleotide likely to have more serious effects on the structure of the protein coded for by that gene?

● Because all of the triplets following the mutation will change and hence the amino acid structure of the resulting protein will be very different.

Mutations of this type are referred to as **frame shift mutations** and frequently lead to a complete loss of function in the resulting protein.

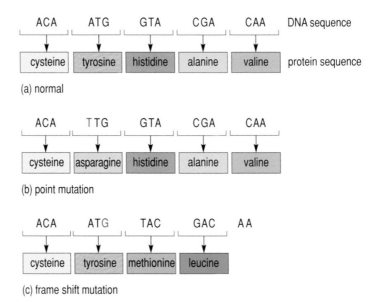

(a) normal

(b) point mutation

(c) frame shift mutation

Figure 1.2 (a) A sequence of DNA bases showing the nucleotide triplets and the amino acids that are coded for by these triplets; (b) a point mutation in which the fourth nucleotide of the sequence has mutated from adenine to thymine and, as a result the amino acid asparagine is substituted for tyrosine in the resulting peptide sequence; (c) a frame shift mutation in which the seventh base (the second guanine) has been lost, resulting in a changed amino acid sequence from this point onwards.

Case Report 1.1 Sickle cell anaemia

Thomas is a 36-year-old man of West African descent who has sickle cell anaemia. Most of the time he looks like a healthy person but the disease has meant he has needed to modify his life in a number of ways. At school he found games lessons to be a particular trial because sickle cell anaemia often left him breathless and short of energy, and teachers did not seem to understand this. Thomas now knows precisely what can precipitate a crisis in his condition; for example, swimming is a great challenge since Thomas knows that cold temperatures can cause a sickle cell crisis (see below). He knows that in sickle cell disease the haemoglobin in his blood is different from normal haemoglobin. Although it can still carry oxygen it tends to crystallize when it releases oxygen. This causes the red blood cell to distort into a sickle shape instead of retaining its normal doughnut shape (Figure 1.3). In turn, this sickle shape disrupts the smooth flow of blood into the narrower vessels, leading to blockages. It is these blockages that are known as sickle cell crises, and they can lead to damaged internal organs as well as being very painful. A crisis usually requires hospitalization and in some cases a blood transfusion is needed. Repeated crises can lead to liver, lung, kidney damage and other medical conditions. Unfortunately, in his late twenties, Thomas suffered kidney failure which resulted in him being admitted to intensive care and having to be off work for many weeks.

In some respects, Thomas finds the unpredictability of his condition one of the most difficult things to cope with. He knows that dehydration, infection, fever, a sudden change in temperature, alcohol and emotional stress are all factors that can precipitate a

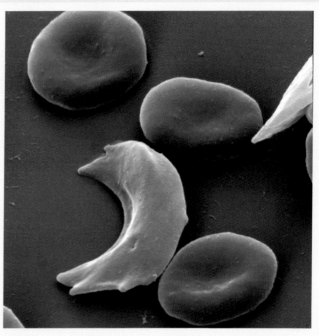

Figure 1.3 Photographs of normal and sickled red blood cells.

crisis. To ward these off, Thomas takes special measures. For example, he knows he must keep warm at all times and in the winter wears hat, scarf, gloves and a thick coat as soon as the weather becomes chilly. He also knows that he must drink plenty of fluids, not overexert himself and take plenty of rest. He feels great tiredness from time to time and takes analgesics frequently to counter the pain he often experiences. For Thomas, this pain is most often located in his legs and lower back. Although there is no cure Thomas knows there is plenty that he can do to reduce the risk of crisis, and he makes certain he has regular hospital check-ups to keep his condition manageable.

1.2.2 Meiosis: independent assortment and recombination

Mutations represent the only way in which new genetic information can be incorporated into the genome (the total genetic information of the organism – Book 1, Section 2.6). However, the process of cell division that gives rise to gametes in sexually reproducing mammals provides two ways in which the existing pool of alleles in a population can be re-assorted into new combinations. Humans are **diploid** organisms in which each cell contains two matching but non-identical (*homologous*) copies of each of the 23 chromosomes, as shown in Figure 2.12 of Book 1. Our gametes (sperm or eggs, **spermatozoa** or **ova**) have just a single copy of each chromosome and are described as **haploid**. Thus,

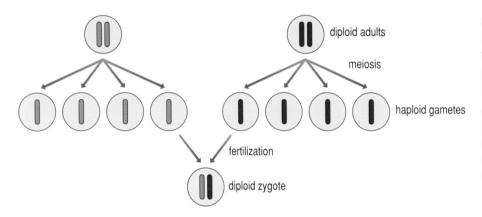

Figure 1.4 The alternation of diploid and haploid stages in a mammalian life cycle. The process begins with two diploid individuals (one male and one female) who then generate haploid gametes. Fertilization allows haploid gametes to fuse and produce the next generation of diploid individuals.

sexual reproduction in mammals involves an alternation between the diploid adult and its haploid gametes, which then fuse during fertilization (a process known as *syngamy*) to generate new diploid offspring (Figure 1.4). These offspring also have 23 homologous chromosome pairs; one chromosome of each pair being derived from the mother, and one from the father.

Figure 1.5 shows a generalized version of the process of meiosis which produces the gametes. In the first stage each chromosome replicates and two individual strands become visible (Figure 1.5a). Matching, or *homologous*, chromosomes pair up (Figure 1.5b). Once the chromosomes are precisely lined up in their pairs, crossing over, or *recombination* of gene variants (alleles) on individual chromosomes, can take place (Figure 1.5c–d). This is a random process in which the individual chromosomes break and rejoin in such a way that homologous portions of the chromosomes are exchanged between members of a pair. The consequence, shown in Figure 1.5e, is that the resulting chromosomes contain novel combinations of alleles deriving from the paternal and maternal chromosomes that originally gave rise to that individual. The cell now divides for the first time (Figure 1.5f) and it is at this point that *independent assortment* takes place. The critical point is that individual chromosome pairs assort independently at this stage. Thus the division might result in one mostly paternal (blue) chromosome A being allocated to the same cell as a mostly maternal (red) chromosome B (or *vice versa*) as is shown in Figure 1.5f. However, it would be equally possible that the mostly maternal (red) copies of chromosomes A and B would end up together, with the mostly paternal (blue) copies in the other cell. Remember that we show only two pairs of chromosomes in this figure but in reality humans have 23 pairs of chromosomes. Thus, the most extreme example of the consequence of independent assortment would be to have *all* 23 of the maternal chromosomes in one daughter cell and *all* 23 of the paternal chromosomes in the other daughter cell by the end of division 1 of meiosis. Even with a rather less dramatic asymmetry of parental chromosomes one can see the basis for a grandparent failing to see any signs of a 'likeness to my family' in a grandchild!

Figure 1.5g then shows the beginning of the second cell division of meiosis which results in the formation of haploid gametes that contain only one copy of each chromosome.

DIVISION I OF MEIOSIS

(a) Chromosomes appear. They have replicated so each shows as two strands. Red chromosomes have been inherited from the mother, blue chromosomes from the father.

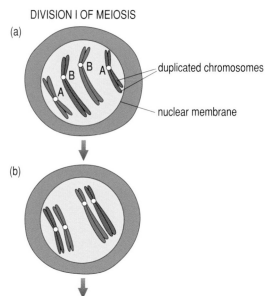

duplicated chromosomes

nuclear membrane

Figure 1.5 A generalized diagram of meiosis and recombination showing the sequence of events for just two pairs of chromosomes; in reality humans have 23 pairs of chromosomes.

(b) Chromosomes pair up: the two chromosomes A form one pair, the two chromosomes B form another.

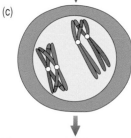

DIVISION II OF MEIOSIS

(c) The strands cross over and exchange material.

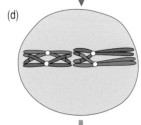

(g) Beginning of division II. (Only one of the two cells of stage (f) is shown here – the upper one.)

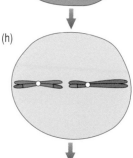

(d) Nuclear membrane disappears and chromosomes line up at equator of cell.

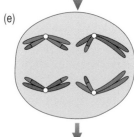

(h) Nuclear envelope breaks down and chromosomes align themselves at equator.

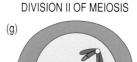

(e) Chromosomes pull away and move to opposite poles of the cell.

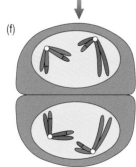

(i) Separation occurs. Single chromosomes move to opposite poles.

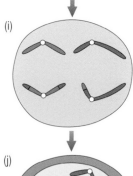

(f) Nuclear membranes develop around both sets of chromosomes and cell divides into two. Each cell contains one-half of the genetic material possessed by the cell shown in (a).

(j) New nuclear membranes form and cell divides into two. This is the haploid state; chromosome A′ does not have a pair, neither does B′. They are labelled A′ and B′ to indicate that due to recombination they are not necessarily identical to A and B shown in (a).

In this way, sexual reproduction provides two ways of using the variation within the gene pool of a population. It randomly assorts the maternal and paternal chromosomes of any one individual into that individual's gametes and also, through recombination, generates individual chromosomes with new mixtures of alleles. As a consequence, it is likely that evolution by natural selection will occur more rapidly in species that reproduce sexually simply because natural selection has more variation on which to work. Recombination requires a complex set of enzymes to break and then rejoin the DNA, and it turns out that these enzymes are also found in simple organisms that do not show meiosis or use sexual reproduction. The function of the enzymes in these organisms is to repair DNA damage within chromosomes, which is in fact a function that they retain in all species.

Occasional errors in pairing and recombination during meiosis may provide a further source of variation in the genome. Sometimes recombination occurs after incorrect pairing of homologous chromosomes. A consequence may be the production of a new chromosome in which some genes are either missing or duplicated. When genes are duplicated in this way they may, in successive generations, begin to evolve separately. For example, one copy of the gene may gain a point mutation while the other copy remains unchanged. It may then turn out that the different copies produce proteins with slightly different properties. Such a mechanism has probably produced the range of different haemoglobins in different species, or even within species. For example, in humans, adult and fetal haemoglobin have slightly different properties in relation to oxygen transport. Fetal haemoglobin binds oxygen more effectively than the adult form and hence oxygen tends to dissociate from the adult form at the placenta and instead binds to the fetal form (Book 3, Section 3.2.4). The difference in this property of the two haemoglobins arises because the fetus produces a gamma globin, rather than the beta globin that is synthesized after birth. The two proteins, and hence the genes that code for them, are closely related but distinct, and probably originally arose as a consequence of gene duplication. The embryo produces yet another closely related haemoglobin for the first 12 weeks.

In addition to these changes within single chromosomes, it also possible for the pairing and separation of chromosomes to proceed incorrectly so that the resulting gametes have additional or missing copies of one or more chromosomes. After fertilization, the resulting zygote will not have the normal diploid number of chromosomes, and this condition is referred to as **aneuploidy**. It is even possible for gametes to be formed in which there are two copies of every chromosome rather than the usual single copy. The resulting zygote will have three copies of every chromosome and is described as *triploid*. A triploid or *tetraploid* (four copies of every chromosome) zygote can also arise as a result of fertilization of an **ovum** by more than one sperm. These last two possibilities, as we shall see in the next section, are not compatible with human development, though they are quite common in some other species of animals and plants, where, as keen gardeners may know, they can give rise to exotic and highly prized blooms.

1.2.3 Meiosis and human reproduction

In Chapter 4 you will see how physiological processes involved in the process of sperm and egg production ultimately lead to the production of a healthy human baby. Since meiosis is central to this process, and, in evolutionary terms, is so ancient, you might imagine that it hardly ever gives rise to problems that affect human fertility. In fact this seems to be far from true!

It is well known that, following fertilization, the early development of an embryo does not always result in an established pregnancy. Embryos do not **implant** (attach to the mother's tissues) until at least 7 days after fertilization so these pre-implantation embryos can be recovered by uterine lavage, a technique used in the context of human fertility treatment, in which fluid is flushed through the uterus. Research findings from *in vitro* fertilization (IVF) clinics have provided insights into the incidence of abnormalities in these early embryos. (The term *in vitro* literally means 'in glass' indicating that fertilization has taken place outside the body in the laboratory glassware, hence the popular name of 'test-tube baby' for babies born as a result of IVF. Clearly the whole of their development did not take place in the laboratory! Chapter 4 gives more details.) Only about 20–40% of embryos produced *in vitro* develop into **blastocysts**, an early stage of fetal development in which the embryo is a hollow ball of cells. Furthermore, many embryos produced *in vitro* have chromosome abnormalities including aneuploidy and structural rearrangements in which part of a chromosome has broken off and joined up to another chromosome. However, these findings are no different from those observed following uterine lavage of naturally fertilized embryos.

It has been known since the 1970s that spontaneously aborted embryos have a high incidence of chromosome anomalies, currently estimated at 40–60%. Although such spontaneous abortions can be emotionally upsetting, the high rates of loss of embryos with chromosomal abnormalities can also be regarded as contributing to a woman's chance of having a healthy baby. Table 1.1 is a summary of chromosomal abnormalities found in spontaneous abortuses and in **neonates** (new-born babies). The commonest type of chromosome abnormality is aneuploidy. Figure 1.6 (overleaf) demonstrates the consequences of this type of error during formation of the gametes in meiosis.

Table 1.1 Incidence of chromosome abnormalities in spontaneously aborted human embryos. (*Note*: See text overleaf for explanation of unfamiliar terms.)

Description of chromosomal abnormality	% aborted embryos	% surviving to birth
Triploidy: 3 complete sets of chromosomes	12–15	<0.01
Tetraploidy: 4 complete sets of chromosomes	3–5	<0.01
Sex chromosome aneuploidy: 3 sex chromosomes	<1	>99
Sex chromosome aneuploidy: 1 sex chromosome	10	<1
Autosome aneuploidy: 3 of one or two autosomes (e.g. 3 copies of chromosome 21)	20–40	3
Autosome aneuploidy: 1 chromosome only of one or two autosomes (e.g. only 1 copy of chromosome 21)	1	None
Structural rearrangement between chromosomes, e.g. a piece of one chromosome is detached and joins up to another chromosome, so two abnormal chromosomes result.	2–3	35

Figure 1.6 (a) Non-separation of one pair of homologous chromosome during meiosis. For simplicity only two pairs of chromosomes are drawn. The first stages of meiosis proceed as shown in Figure 1.5a–c. Figure 1.6a shows the chromosome pairs lining up in the middle of the cell. The members of each chromosome pair should move to opposite poles of the cell but this does not happen for one chromosome pair, resulting in an extra chromosome in one of the daughter cells (Figure 1.6b).

First stages of division I of meiosis are as shown in Figure 1.5a–c

DIVISION II OF MEIOSIS

Nuclear membrane disappears and chromosomes line up at equator of cell.

(a)

Division II of meiosis now proceeds as shown in Figure 1.5

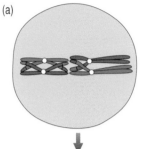

Chromosomes pull away and move to opposite poles of the cell but one homologous pair remains together.

(b)

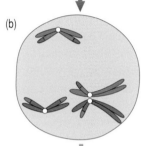

Nuclear membranes develop around both sets of chromosomes and cell divides into two, but now daughter cell D1 has only one chromosome, and daughter cell D2 has three.

(c)

D1

D2

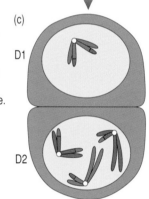

Figure 1.6a represents the stage of meiosis in which the pairs of chromosomes line up at the equator of the cell. (It is identical to Figure 1.5d.) Next one member of each pair should migrate to opposite ends of the cell as shown in Figure 1.5e but in this case (Figure 1.6b) both chromosomes of one pair have migrated to the same pole of the cell.

● What is the effect on the chromosome numbers of the two daughter cells in the first division of meiosis, if one pair of homologous chromosomes remains together instead of separating?

● One of the daughter cells has an extra chromosome and the other daughter cell lacks one chromosome.

Figure 1.6c shows the two daughter cells. Now the second division of meiosis begins in each of the two daughter cells, D1 and D2. In the second meiotic division, each of the daughter cells divides again.

● How many chromosomes will be present in the two daughter cells of D1?

● One in each; there is a red chromosome missing.

● How many chromosomes would you expect in the two daughter cells of D2?

● There will be three in each, because there are two copies of the red chromosome and one copy of the blue.

Therefore there will be two daughter cells, which are the gametes, with three chromosomes and two daughter cells with just one chromosome. For humans that originate from such abnormal gametes, an extra chromosome would mean a total of 47 chromosomes instead of 46. Aneuploidies resulting from fertilization of an egg with a missing **autosomal chromosome** are usually incompatible with further development (Table 1.1). (Autosomal refers to all chromosomes other than the X and Y sex-determining chromosomes.)

● If a sperm with a normal genotype, including one chromosome 21, fertilizes an egg that has two chromosome 21s, how many copies of chromosome 21 will the zygote nucleus contain?

● The zygote will contain three copies of chromosome 21. [This condition is described as trisomy 21.]

Although aneuploidies may arise as a result of an extra chromosome in either the sperm or egg, the incidence of aneuploidies in eggs is known to increase with age in women, and sharply so beyond the maternal age of 40 years.

● Baby girls are born with their full complement of eggs arrested in an early part of the first meiotic division (Figure 1.5). Estimate the age range of eggs that are ovulated (i.e. released each menstrual cycle) from puberty to the onset of menopause.

● Assuming that ovulation begins at or shortly after puberty and ends at the menopause, ovulated eggs can be from about 14–50 years old.

As eggs age they are more susceptible to errors during meiosis, especially aneuploidies. As Table 1.1 shows, very few chromosome aneuploidies are compatible with life and the embryos often fail to develop sufficiently to implant (attach to the womb). Of those that survive to implantation, many are lost in the first three months of pregnancy. Some rare aneuploidies such as **trisomy 18** (three chromosome 18s; Edward's syndrome) are usually compatible with life but only for about 1–6 days after birth. In contrast, long-term survival of babies with **trisomy 21**, Down's syndrome, is likely. Such babies have three chromosome 21s derived from fertilization of an egg or, more rarely, a sperm, bearing two copies of chromosome 21. Other examples of chromosome aneuploidy compatible with life include those associated with the sex chromosomes X and Y.

● What is the usual sex chromosome genotype for (i) males and (ii) females?

● (i) The usual male genotype is XY, with one copy of an X chromosome derived from the mother and one copy of the Y chromosome derived from the father. (ii) The usual female genotype is XX, with one copy derived from the mother and one from the father (Book 1, Section 2.5.2). Since such individuals have the normal 46 chromosomes they can be described as 46XY and 46XX.

Some women have an XXX sexual genotype; there is no associated pathology and they are fertile. Some male individuals have an extra X chromosome, resulting in the sexual genotype XXY; such men are sometimes said to have **Klinefelter's syndrome**. XXY males frequently live normal lives and are likely to be unaware that they have an extra X chromosome; it is estimated that as many as 1 in 500 males have the XXY genotype (see Case Report 1.2). However, the XXY males are almost always infertile and clinical investigations, including chromosomal studies, may provide the first diagnosis of an XXY genotype for an individual. XXY males may have difficulties in language development that affect their reading and writing ability, and it can be useful for parents to be aware that their child has the XXY genotype so that such specific learning difficulties can be addressed.

Case Report 1.2 Klinefelter's syndrome

James is 32 years old and has been married for four years. He and Beena, his wife, want to have children but Beena has not conceived. As a result of fertility investigations, James was diagnosed as having Klinefelter's syndrome. This syndrome was first outlined by Dr Harry Klinefelter in 1942 and is estimated to affect 1 in 500 to 1 in 1000 male live births. Men with Klinefelter's syndrome have an extra sex chromosome giving 47XXY instead of the more usual 46XY. As James has read, women usually inherit two X chromosomes, one from each parent. Men inherit an X chromosome from their mothers and a Y chromosome from their fathers. However, the meiosis that occurs in the cells destined to become eggs and sperm occasionally gives rise to an egg with two X chromosomes or a sperm with both an X and Y. There are two ways of producing an XXY male. Either an XY sperm fertilizes an X egg or a Y sperm fertilizes an XX egg. There are other less common variations such as 48XXXY or 49XXXXY. There is also a mosaic type where some body cells have the usual 46XY complement and others have the Klinefelter 47XXY complement.

James was surprised when the cause of infertility was identified; he had never heard of the syndrome before. As James learnt more about the syndrome, he became aware that although it is probably one of the most common chromosome variations, it is not well known to the general public or even to many in the health care professions. Furthermore, no two people with the syndrome are the same. The only common factors are

that men have an extra chromosome and have undeveloped testes and hence are usually infertile. When puberty occurs the testes remain small and this persists into adult life. Some people with the syndrome may be taller than average, but not excessively so. James understands that men with Klinefelter's syndrome can have less body hair than average or it can even fail to develop. Men with the syndrome can also have a pear-shape weight distribution and develop breasts. However, James has none of these signs though he does have long limbs compared to his body and big feet, signs that can be indicative of the syndrome. James has read that boys who exhibit many of the signs of Klinefelter's can find themselves teased at school because of the physical characteristics they develop and this can in turn lead to behavioural problems. James experienced none of the very obvious physical or psychological effects and so, alongside many others with the syndrome, has lived his life unaware of the extra chromosome.

James had read that many characteristics, but not height and infertility, can be relieved by testosterone replacement therapy given from puberty onwards. The level is determined by a GP and an endocrinologist since to some extent some Klinefelter's syndrome males can make their own testosterone. However, Beena and James have been informed that there are very few cases, at present, of men with Klinefelter's who have been able to father children. Beena and James are now seeking further specialist advice on this matter.

● Individuals with an XXY genotype have a male phenotype, whereas individuals with an XX genotype have a female phenotype. What does this suggest about the genetic basis of sex determination in humans?

● It suggests there is a gene, or genes, on the Y chromosome, that when activated, leads to male-typical development.

In fact one important sex-determining gene of this type, known as the sex-determining gene of the Y chromosome (*SRY*) has been clearly identified, first in mice, and more recently in humans. This gene is activated before the 6th week of pregnancy, though, obviously, only in a male fetus. The protein product of *SRY* influences the tissue that will develop into either a testis or an ovary. At this early stage of development the tissue is referred to as the *indifferent gonad*. When the SRY protein is present, the tissue begins to develop as a testis and immediately secretes the steroid hormone testosterone. The testosterone that circulates in the fetus then pushes further development, especially of genitalia, but also other structures, including the brain, in a 'male-like' direction. As development proceeds, the testis becomes inactive, and remains so until puberty when testosterone secretion resumes again. In the absence of *SRY* activation, in a female embryo, the indifferent gonad develops instead into an ovary. Of course, many other genes are involved in the development and proper functioning of testes, ovaries and the other organs required for reproduction but *SRY* does have a critical early role in determining the direction in which sexual development will proceed.

1.2.4 Gene–environment interactions

The phenotype of an organism is, as the examples in the previous sections demonstrate, strongly influenced by its genotype. Whether hair colour is blond, red or black will depend on the presence or absence of particular enzymes in the hair follicle, and this, in turn, will depend on the particular set of alleles possessed by that individual. However, in many cases, and especially for more complex behavioural traits, inheritance cannot be attributed this simply. Many individual genes may influence one aspect of the phenotype. In addition, environmental variables may influence the phenotype. A wide variety of factors contribute to the environment experienced by an individual, from simple physical factors, such as temperature, through to complex features such as the family or social background.

It may be tempting to suppose that the total variability in a particular trait can be divided into two parts, one genetic and the other environmental, which then simply add up to determine the phenotype. In fact it is very hard to partition the variability in this simple way. Often a particular phenotype will require both the appropriate genotype and a particular set of environmental features before it is likely to develop.

● Can you think of an earlier example from the course of this type of interaction?

● Phenylketonuria (Book 1, Case Report 1.1) is a disease that results from an inability to metabolize the amino acid phenylalanine. It results from a single gene defect and leads to brain damage and behavioural dysfunction. However, if the amino acid is removed from the diet then the effects on brain development will be avoided.

Many other diseases have this general characteristic. For example, individuals who have a deficiency of the enzyme α-1-antitrypsin are very much more likely to develop a serious lung disease, emphysema, if they smoke cigarettes. The normal function of the antitrypsin is to protect body tissues, especially the lungs, from substances released by white cells as they respond to inflammation or infection (Book 1, Section 2.10.2). Smoking strongly promotes these inflammatory responses in the lung, and this explains how the combination of the genetic change and the environmental variable makes emphysema very much more probable.

For behavioural traits, complex interactions between genotype may occur across generations. Think of a musical family like that of Johann Sebastian Bach. It may be that the large number of talented musicians in the subsequent two generations of his family was specifically influenced by their genotype. However, Bach also provided an environment for his family which would have been quite different to that of most 16th century North German families. So even if some aspect of his children's genotype favoured musical ability, the environment in which the children were raised would surely have greatly exaggerated this tendency. In many other cases, such exceptional ability will appear in one generation only, and the processes of recombination and independent assortment may provide a partial explanation for this outcome, in that favourable combinations of alleles can be lost.

Summary of Section 1.2

1   Humans are variable, in part because they are genetically diverse but also because no two individuals share exactly the same environment.

2   Genetic variability ultimately depends on changes (mutations) in the genetic material (DNA).

3   Some mutations, including many point mutations, produce only slight changes in protein function but others, including frame shift mutations, may produce complete loss of function.

4   Recombination and independent assortment of genetic material from paternal and maternal chromosomes, which occurs during meiosis, can enhance genetic variability.

5   Chromosome abnormalities caused by errors in meiosis, e.g. aneuploidies, account for the loss of a relatively high proportion of embryos in early pregnancy.

6   Attempts to divide individual variability into genetic and environmental components are difficult from both a theoretical and a practical perspective.

1.3 Genes, environment and the causes of obesity

In this section we will look at the ways in which environmental and genetic factors interact to produce the diversity that is characteristic of humans and other species. We will use variation in human body weight and changes in the incidence of obesity, first discussed in Book 1, Chapter 3, as a case study.

1.3.1 Ron revisited

In Book 1 (Case Report 3.1) you met Ron. Ron is 59 years old, has a BMI of 31 and a central obesity ratio of 0.96, indicating that he is moderately obese, with the fat concentrated in his abdomen, rather than his hips. Clearly a number of factors, some environmental, others relating to Ron's age and all interacting with Ron's genetic constitution, may help to provide an explanation. Let's look at some of these factors in a little more detail. It is clear that Ron enjoys a comfortable lifestyle with little exercise and a generous diet. Three cooked meals a day, snacks and the occasional glass of beer might easily generate an energy input of more than 12 000 kJ day^{-1}.

● What is Ron's estimated average requirement (EAR), expressed in kJ day^{-1}?

● This can be calculated from Book 1, Table 3.1. Ron's EAR is 2550 kcal × 4.2 = 10 710 kJ. (4.2 is the correction factor required to transform calories to joules; Book 1, Section 3.2.2.)

You might wonder, given the emphasis earlier in the course on physiological systems providing homeostatic control (e.g. Book 1, Section 2.4), why Ron doesn't feel permanently sated, leading to a reduction in his food intake and body weight. Studies with volunteers living in a laboratory environment in which food intake and energy output could be continuously monitored over several weeks provide a partial answer to this paradox.

1.3.2 Experimental studies of energy balance

The energy that a human takes in, primarily in food or nutritive fluids, has to be balanced by the energy lost in various ways. Some energy is used to maintain basic metabolic processes, some in physical activity while the remainder is lost as heat, or in the faeces or urine. If energy input and output do not balance, then the residue must either result in a loss or a gain in body weight.

One way of estimating these energy fluxes is to use the technique of *whole room indirect calorimetry*. Volunteers live on their own in a small suite of rooms which are sealed from the outside environment. The room can also contain exercise equipment. Food and water are provided through an airlock, and the exact amounts of carbon dioxide produced and oxygen used are measured. It is then possible to calculate an overall energy budget for each individual.

In one experiment of this type, participants were divided into three groups, each group receiving a diet of different fat content (Poppitt and Prentice, 1996). The other constituents of the diet, which were mainly protein and carbohydrate, were varied in such a way as to keep the overall energy density of the diets constant.

● What is the energy density of a diet?

● The number of calories (or joules) in a standard quantity (often 100 g) of that food (Book 1, Section 3.2.2).

The participants in this experiment were not aware that their diets were being manipulated in this way. In practical terms this kind of manipulation is achieved

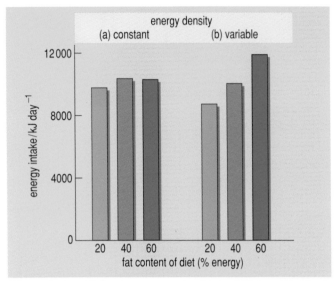

Figure 1.7 Voluntary energy intake and dietary energy density in energy-manipulated diets. In (a) the other dietary constituents were manipulated so that the overall energy density remained constant as the proportion of fat was increased. In (b) no change was made in other dietary constituents as fat was added and as a consequence the overall energy density of the diet increased.

by, for example, substituting fat for carbohydrate within a yogurt while, at the same time, ensuring that the sensory characteristics (e.g. taste, smell and feel) do not change.

The results of this experiment are shown in Figure 1.7(a).

● How did the voluntary energy intake of the participants vary as a function of the fat content of the diets when energy density is constant?

◑ The overall result was straightforward: the energy intake of the volunteers hardly varies as a function of the amount of fat in the diet.

The apparent difference between the 20% and 40% groups was not significant. In addition there was no significant change in body weight over the experimental period of a few days.

In a second experiment the participants were again divided into three groups. Now each group received a diet in which the fat content had been covertly manipulated so as to *vary* the total energy density. One group received a diet which was relatively low fat and low energy, in a second group it was relatively normal whereas the third group received an energy-dense, high-fat diet. Other factors, such as the palatability of the foods provided, were again held constant. Surprisingly, the participants in the different experimental groups ate about the same number of grams of food each day regardless of its energy content.

● Look at Figure 1.7(b). What was the consequence of this behaviour for the energy intake of the participants?

◑ The consequence was that participants in the high energy density and fat content group had a higher energy intake than those in the groups provided with foods of lower energy density and fat content.

One result of these different energy intakes was that participants in the high-fat group increased in weight during the study period whereas those on the low-fat group lost weight. Taken together, the results of these experiments suggest that humans don't respond very accurately to changes in the energy density of their diet especially when their diet is very high in fat!

Detailed calculations based on these experiments suggest that excess consumption of about 3×10^4 kJ of fat had generated about 100 g of adipose tissue by the end of the experimental period. A hamburger and french fries from one major fast food retailer is shown on their website as containing 2.92×10^4 kJ [*] with a high proportion of that energy being in the form of fat. There is a good deal of evidence to suggest that dietary fat, protein and carbohydrate may differ in the degree to which they can induce satiety – that rather pleasant feeling of satisfaction and

[*]Big Mac ™ and regular fries are shown as 699 kC (kcal) with an energy density of 494 kC per 100 g. 1 joule is approx 0.239 kC, giving a total energy content of 2924 kJ and an energy density of 2066 kJ per 100g (McDonalds, 2005).

fullness that we experience at the end of a meal. Carbohydrate and protein, when matched in terms of energy content, are very much more effective in enhancing satiety than is fat. You can now easily imagine how regular consumption of energy dense, high-fat foods might translate into increased body weight.

Another dietary factor that may be related to the increased incidence of obesity is the use of fructose derived from corn (high-fructose corn syrup) as a sweetener in soft drinks. Fructose is a simple sugar, like glucose, but differs from it in several important ways. Fructose can be absorbed by cells in the absence of insulin, and is also a poor signal for insulin release. Once in a cell it can be very easily metabolized into glycerol, one of the building blocks for fat (see Box 1.1 on Adipose tissue, which should be read after completing study of Section 1.3.6). Bray (2004) has pointed out the very close parallel between increases in the use of high-fructose corn syrup in the food industry and the incidence of obesity in North America. Of course, soft drinks sweetened in this way are frequently consumed together with the kinds of energy-dense, high-fat foods that we discussed in the last few paragraphs, so it will not be easy to disentangle the effects of these two factors. Looking at the data as a natural scientific experiment we might say that the effects of energy-dense, high-fat foods, and of soft drinks sweetened with corn syrup, on the incidence of obesity are confounded together.

Collect the wrappers of some typical snack foods. Look at the dietary information. How effective are they likely to be at inducing satiety? What contribution might they make to total daily energy intake? People often feel that a savoury snack (e.g. crisps) might be healthier than a sweet snack (e.g. chocolate). Does the dietary information that you have just collected support this idea?

1.3.3 Obesity – an evolutionary perspective

If you were now to take a broader biological approach to the data discussed in the previous section you might still be puzzled. Excess body weight leads to a variety of diseases, including diabetes, osteoarthritis and so on – surely this must reduce overall biological fitness.

●   What is biological fitness?

●   The formal definition (Book 1, Section 1.4.2) is 'lifetime reproductive success'. It can be estimated by measuring the number of offspring (or perhaps even grandchildren!) left by an individual relative to other members of that population.

So why are we, as a species, apparently so unresponsive to the potential reduction in fitness that may result from obesity? Why has natural selection not equipped us with satiety mechanisms that are tuned to the types of nutrients found in our diet? A speculative answer to this question is provided by Prentice and Jebb (2003). They suggest that the critical point to consider is the environment in which our evolutionary ancestors lived. Genetic and fossil evidence suggests that our species, *Homo sapiens*, evolved in Africa, around 200 000–120 000 years ago, from an ancient *Homo* species, which had a hunter–gatherer lifestyle. Since then, for most of the time, humans have also been hunter–gatherers, until about 12 000 years ago, when subsistence farming became established. Both the hunter–gatherer and the subsistence farming diets have a much lower energy density than those available in many societies in the developed world. Even today some groups of subsistence farmers exist on diets with an average energy density of about 500 kJ per 100 g, which is only a quarter of the value for a typical fast food meal. Although the diets of other primates species, e.g. chimpanzees, are highly variable, their energy density and fat content are also very much lower than that characteristic of present industrialized societies. Thus our apparent failure to adapt may be because our distant ancestors were not exposed to diets of high energy density and we therefore don't have the appropriate physiological and behavioural responses to such foods.

The idea that humans are best adapted to an environment that is quite different from that in which we now live was first discussed by the child psychologist John Bowlby in 1969 when he referred to our 'Environment of Evolutionary Adaptedness' (EAA). This concept has become very influential in both human behavioural ecology and evolutionary psychology. However, the concept also has its critics because it is very difficult to get unambiguous evidence about exactly what kind of environment our EAA might have been. Prentice and Jebb (2003) suggest that modern day subsistence farmers in Gambia may provide a good model for the kind of diet available during much of our evolutionary past. However, it is likely that early humans lived in a wide variety of environments and that different populations consumed very different types of diet. Even in recent times, hunter–gatherer and subsistence farming populations show tremendous variety in their food sources.

● From your general knowledge, suggest some examples of this type of variety.

◐ The traditional diet of Inuit Indians living in Northern Canada consists almost entirely of protein and fat derived from the seals and salmon that are abundant there. The traditional diet of Masai warriors is also very high in animal fat and yet is not associated with high levels of either obesity or heart disease.

Several alternative, though not mutually exclusive, mechanisms to account for some cases of obesity involve the possibility that some of our ancestors might have had adaptive responses to nutritional shortages. One of the most interesting of these explanations is known as the **'thrifty phenotype' hypothesis** (Ozanne and Hales, 2002); it suggests that poor fetal nutrition leads to adaptive changes in physiology that prepare an adult for a life of poor nutrition (Figure 1.8). However, if poor fetal nutrition is followed by good nutrition in later life then the consequences may include obesity and type 2 diabetes. Evidence to support this idea comes from studies of individuals who were born at the end of a severe famine that occurred in the Netherlands towards the end of World War II – the Dutch Hunger Winter. Pregnant women who were affected by the famine tended to have children of lower birth weight than women who were unaffected by the famine. However, the affected children, as adults, were more likely to be obese and suffer from type 2 diabetes. By contrast, studies of the children of pregnant women in sub-Saharan Africa who also suffered from famine both *in utero* and as adults showed no increase in diabetes. Instead, not surprisingly, they continued to be thin and well adapted to a life of relatively low calorie intake.

Recent studies of monozygotic (identical) twins in Denmark suggest that these effects are a direct result of fetal nutrition and do not depend on genetic differences between individuals. Where identical twins do differ in birth weight, it is the twin with the lighter birth weight who is at greater risk of obesity and diabetes as an adult.

● Why should it be the lighter twin that is most at risk of obesity and diabetes?

◐ Monozygotic twins have identical genotypes so it must be differences in their environment that have led to differences in birth weight. Although they have the same mother and lie in the same womb, one must have been less well nourished. The thrifty phenotype hypothesis would predict that physiological changes had occurred in the lighter twin who would now be better adapted for a life of poor nutrition. As with the children born after the Dutch Hunger Winter, these Danish twins are likely to be well nourished, a situation for which they are not best adapted.

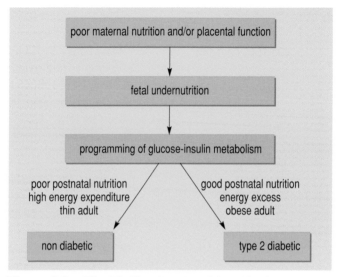

Figure 1.8   The 'thrifty phenotype' hypothesis.

This ability to vary or 'programme' adult physiology as a consequence of early life experiences may be a general feature in mammals since exactly the same responses to fetal malnutrition can be obtained in laboratory rats.

1.3.4 Obesity and brain reward systems

Very palatable foods, especially those high in fat and carbohydrate may be potent stimuli for neural pathways in the brain. Direct evidence for this idea has been found in recent studies of non-human animals. For example, it is known that many types of both natural (i.e. food, sex) and drug (e.g. cocaine or amphetamine, opiates, nicotine) rewards are able to stimulate activity within a brain pathway that innervates the ventral striatum at the base of the forebrain (Figure 1.9). These structures lie within the cerebral hemispheres (Book 2, Section 1.4.1). The nerve cells that make up this pathway, which is called the *mesolimbic dopamine projection*, use dopamine as their neurotransmitter. Thus, when a rat eats a highly palatable and very sweet breakfast cereal there is an almost immediate increase in the release of dopamine within the ventral striatum. Other foods high in fat and carbohydrate are known to activate the same brain system.

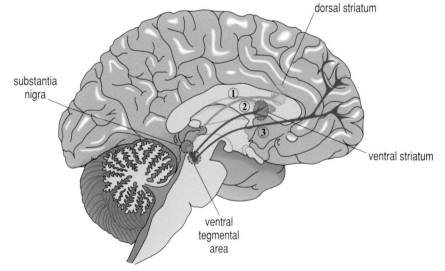

Figure 1.9   Human dopamine projections. (1) The nigrostriatal projection, which is concerned with movement (see Book 2, Section 1.10 for the role of dopaminergic neurons in initiating movement). (2) and (3) The mesolimbic dopamine projection, which is involved in reward-related functions.

There is preliminary evidence that the same pathway may be involved in human responses to food-related cues. Recently Nora Volkow and her colleagues (Wang et al., 2001) used brain imaging techniques to visualize dopamine receptor availability in the brains of both normal weight and morbidly obese individuals (Figure 1.10a). They found significantly lowered dopamine receptor availability in the ventral striatum of the obese individuals.

● If dopamine receptor availability is lowered, what might be the effect on the functioning of the mesolimbic dopamine projection?

● When the mesolimbic dopamine projection is stimulated to release dopamine, the cells in the ventral striatum will receive a smaller signal than usual because they have fewer receptors available to 'pick up' the neurotransmitters.

● The lower of the two sets of images in Figure 1.10a shows brain metabolic activity in obese and in control individuals. Why was it important to measure brain metabolic activity in this study?

● The reduced dopamine receptor availability might have been a reflection of a much more general change in brain function. The absence of any difference in brain metabolic activity suggests that the change in dopamine receptor availability is a quite specific effect.

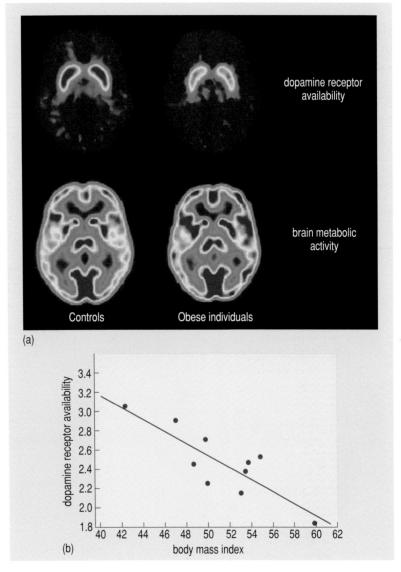

(a)

(b)

Figure 1.10 Measurements of the relationship between dopamine receptor availability and obesity. (a) The upper pair of images show dopamine receptor availability in control and obese participants. Note the clear difference between them. The lower pair of images show brain metabolic activity (see Book 2, Figure 1.1). Note that there is no difference between them. (b) The relationship between brain dopamine receptor availability and the degree of obesity. You do not need to be aware of the measurement units for dopamine receptor availability.

● Use Figure 1.10b to describe the relationship between dopamine receptor availability and the degree of obesity.

◐ The extent to which dopamine receptor availability was reduced was directly proportional to the degree of obesity; the more obese the individuals, the fewer the numbers of receptors available.

Volkow and her colleagues reasoned that the lowered dopamine receptor availability might generate pathological increases in eating as a compensatory response. Interestingly, similar decreases in dopamine receptor availability have been observed in the brains of people addicted to cocaine. However, in both cases, it is not possible to say whether the lowered dopamine receptor availability was the original cause of a pathological increase in eating, or an adaptive response that occurred only at a later stage.

There is also good evidence for the involvement of cortical areas in our response to the particular sensory characteristics of fat. Rolls and his colleagues (Rolls, 2004), working at Oxford, have used an imaging technique (fMRI) to demonstrate activation of parts of the frontal lobe, including the orbitofrontal and insular cortex, by fat-like stimuli. These two areas receive sensory inputs from the mouth and tongue and also have important connections to the ventral striatum (Figure 1.9).

1.3.5 Obesity and ageing

So, it seems that a part of the explanation for Ron's obesity, and the health problems that have led him to seek medical advice, may relate to the environment in which he is living, and more specifically the diet that he has chosen. It may also be a diet that is especially effective in activating the reward circuits in Ron's brain. However, Ron is also in his later middle age. A longitudinal study of people of this age in the USA suggests that average body weight increases by 1–2 kg per decade in later middle age (He and Baker, 2004).

● Is this observed weight increase necessarily a consequence of age? What other explanation can you suggest?

◐ This observation of increased average body weight might not represent an effect of age – instead it might have resulted from a change in the typical diets of this group of Americans over the 10 year period of the study – perhaps the participants were eating more energy-dense, high-fat food at the end of the study period than at the beginning because of cultural changes within the society within which they lived. As previously mentioned, there may have been changes to the way that the food they were eating has been processed, such as the increased use of corn syrup as a sweetener. This could lead to an altered total energy intake occurring *without* the participants making any obvious changes to their diets.

It certainly is the case that obesity has increased very markedly in both USA (Figure 1.11) and Europe during the last 20 years, and this applies to young as well as older people.

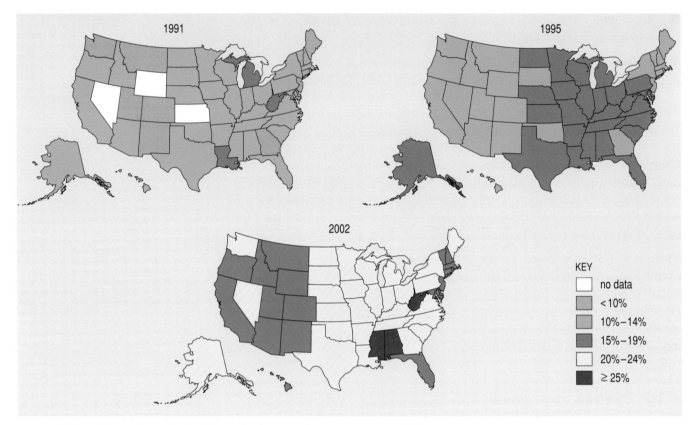

Figure 1.11 Maps of obesity incidence in the USA in 1991, 1995 and 2002.

However, it is also possible that the increase in Ron's weight is due to age-related changes in his behaviour or physiology. Remember that changes in body weight can only occur when energy intake and output differ. There are several reasons why energy expenditure might decrease as we age.

● What suggestions can you make?

● There may be a tendency to exercise less frequently and intensely.

In addition, some of the hormonal changes associated with ageing may tend to reduce basal metabolic rate. For example, the levels of gonadal steroids, including androgens such as testosterone, decrease substantially. Amongst its many effects, testosterone tends to increase metabolic rate and promote production of muscle rather than adipose tissue. So, even in individuals eating the same diet over the period of a decade, there might be a tendency for body weight to increase if food consumption does not drop.

1.3.6 A gene 'for' obesity?

So far we have mostly emphasized the way in which different environmental factors may affect body weight and provide a partial explanation of both individual cases of obesity and the increase in average body weight that has been so clearly documented in both North America and Western Europe during the last two decades. There is also marked individual variability in body weight. For example, any weight between about 58 and 78 kg would be regarded as 'desirable' for a person of height 1.77 m.

● Why might this range of body weight be regarded as desirable for someone with a height of 1.77 m?

● In Book 1 (Table 3.4) you will find the range of BMIs regarded as desirable. The lower end of the desirable range is shown as 18.5, which, when substituted into the formula for the BMI of a person of 1.77 m in height, gives a body weight of 57.96 kg. The upper end of the desirable range is 25, giving a weight of 78.32 kg for persons of this height.

Clearly the actual range of body weights found in human populations is very much greater than the desirable range, and the environmental factors discussed earlier may explain a substantial part of this variation between individuals. But it is also possible that some of this variation depends on specific genetic differences between individuals.

There is considerable evidence to suggest that body weight is heritable to some extent. In a classic study, Albert Stunkard and his colleagues (Stunkard et al., 1986) investigated the relationship between adult body weight of 540 adopted Danish adults and the weights of their biological and adoptive parents. The results were clear cut. There was a strong relationship, which extended from individuals who were very thin through to those who were obese, between the weight of adoptees and the weight of both their biological father and mother. There was no relationship between an adoptee's weight and the weight of either adoptive parent. The idea that variability in body weight may be partly under genetic influence also fits with older studies suggesting that different racial groups may have differing propensities to obesity and type 2 diabetes. In 1962, Neel reviewed data suggesting that certain human populations, including some South Pacific Islanders and North American Indians, may have a genotype that promotes increased fat storage. This genotype represents a survival advantage in times of famine, but can predispose these populations to obesity and type 2 diabetes in typical Westernized societies (see Bindon and Baker, 1997). This is usually known as the **'thrifty genotype' hypothesis**. It is important to note that this hypothesis is not suggested as a universal, or even a common, reason for obesity, but one that applies just to these specific groups.

● How would you characterize the major difference between the thrifty genotype and the thrifty phenotype hypotheses of obesity?

● The thrifty phenotype hypothesis emphasizes the way in which an environmental trigger (poor fetal nutrition) can alter the course of development so as to make obesity more likely when the environment is appropriate. By contrast, the thrifty genotype hypothesis suggests that genetic differences between (racial) groups of individuals makes obesity a more likely consequence in some of those groups when they are exposed to an energy-dense modern diet.

Recent advances in our understanding of both molecular genetics and the hormonal and neurotransmitter controls of feeding have led to specific explanations of some causes of obesity.

Leptin is a hormone produced by adipose tissue that acts on specific nerve cells in the brain stem and hypothalamus to inhibit feeding behaviour (Book 2, Section 3.6.2). It was first identified because a very obese strain of mice was discovered to have a mutation in the gene that codes for leptin. Subsequently, a very small number of human families have been identified in which some individuals also have a mutation in the gene that codes for leptin. These mutations are often of the 'frame-shift' type (see Section 1.2.1) and lead to a complete loss of function in the resulting protein. Humans with such mutations overeat and become very obese. If, as children, attempts are made to restrict their food intake, they may become aggressive and difficult to manage. Treatment with leptin leads to normalization of both appetite and body weight. However, the administration of leptin turns out to be very much less effective in the great majority of morbidly obese individuals. They typically already have very high leptin levels but have lost the normal physiological and behavioural responses to the hormone (Book 2, Section 3.6.2). Thus leptin has not, so far, proved to be the 'magic bullet' that will treat the human obesity epidemic.

In the hypothalamus leptin acts on two groups of nerve cells, both of which influence feeding behaviour but with opposite actions. One set of cells uses neuropeptide Y (NPY) as their neurotransmitter and activation of these cells tends to increase appetite (Figure 1.12). The second set of cells uses α-melanocyte-stimulating hormone (α-MSH) as a neurotransmitter. The α-MSH acts on a subtype of melanocortin receptor known as the MC_4 receptor located on other hypothalamic neurons. Activation of the α-MSH-containing cells is associated with a reduction in feeding behaviour. As you would predict, mice which have been genetically manipulated so that the MC_4 receptor is non-functional overeat and are obese. The functional receptor works by producing a second messenger in the postsynaptic cell when α-MSH is released presynaptically. The production of second messenger is said to be coupled to α-MSH binding.

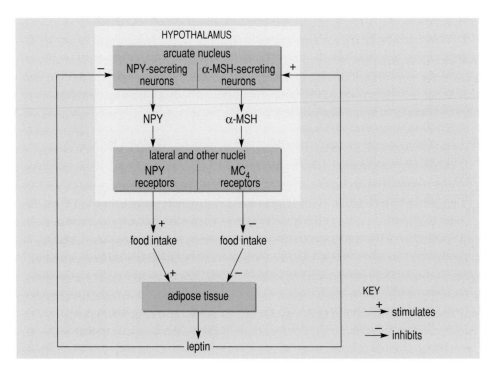

Figure 1.12 Flow chart showing link between action of melanocortins and feeding behaviour.

O'Rahilly and colleagues, working at Cambridge University (Farooqi et al., 2003), have shown that mutations in the human MC_4 receptor may account for about 5% of cases of morbid obesity. A number of different point mutations have been isolated, and are associated with different degrees of obesity. The extent to which each mutation interferes with the coupling between α-MSH binding to the receptor and the production of second messenger has also been determined. There is a good correlation between the two measures. Mutations that are associated with the greatest degree of obesity are those in which coupling is least efficient. So, for these cases, we have a reasonably complete understanding of the way in which single mutations in a gene may lead to changes in a complex behavioural trait such as feeding and then go on to influence the long-term regulation of body weight. But even here the statistical correlation is far from perfect, which means that the genetic variation explains only a part of the individual variation in body weight.

However, in most cases inheritance of obesity is not consistent with a single gene change. If you look back over the different examples that we have discussed, you can see that this is exactly what would be expected. Even though obesity can only reflect greater energy input than output, the imbalance may arise in many different ways. Environmental factors may play an important role, as may early programming of physiology following fetal undernutrition. Genetic factors may also play a critical role in some cases. But to specify the relative importance of these different factors for any particular individual is always likely to be very difficult. However, our increasing understanding of the molecular genetics of obesity can be very positive in specific cases. For example, for those few individuals who are leptin deficient, administration of synthetic leptin provides good treatment. Our increased understanding also makes it clear that to label young individuals with this type of deficiency as gluttons who lack self control, and to characterize their parents as inadequate for failing to control their child's diet and weight is completely inappropriate.

You could now read Box 1.1 on Adipose Tissue or, if you prefer, it can be read after completing study of Section 1.3.

1.3.7 Treatments for obesity

At this point you may be wondering what the range of studies that we have examined might suggest in terms of treatment for obesity. As you have seen, weight gain essentially arises from an imbalance of energy supply and energy expenditure. Therefore it is not surprising that dieting (restriction of energy input) and exercise (increased energy output) are recommended both to reduce body weight and also for their additional health benefits. However, even a quick survey of the research literature makes it clear that dieting is not very effective in the medium or long term as a method of reducing body weight. People find it hard to be compliant with a particular diet, and are also poor at simply recalling what they have eaten. Thus, food diaries are a notoriously inaccurate way of estimating an individual's total food intake. In addition, reduction of food intake, especially with a low-fat diet, may be associated with a depression of metabolic rate that restricts the actual amount of weight that is lost.

Box 1.1   Adipose tissue

In this chapter, and elsewhere in the course, there have been many references to adipose tissue. You probably have a sense of a rather inert (and, perhaps, hard to shift!) tissue acting as a long-term energy store, but this is only a small part of the story.

Adipose tissue consists of individual fat cells (adipocytes (Figure 1.13)) together with connective tissue, a rich blood supply that is shared with adjacent tissues, and innervation from the sympathetic nervous system. The adipocytes are large, clear cells containing stored lipids. The volume of individual adipocytes varies markedly, perhaps as much as tenfold, as adult humans become more or less obese. Mature adipocytes do not divide but differentiate from very much smaller cells known as pre-adipocytes. The number of adipocytes in an adult is influenced by nutrition in fetal and pre-adult life.

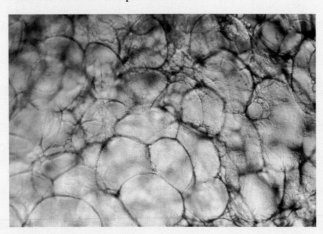

Figure 1.13 Light micrograph of an intact fragment of human adipose tissue.

Adipocytes are often concentrated into fat depots which are characteristic of both species (e.g. a camel's humps) and gender (e.g. a human female's breasts). However, subcutaneous, intramuscular and intra-abdominal fat depots are found in most mammals. The paunch, characteristic of many primates, including our own species, is formed from a thickening of the outer wall of the abdomen. These various fat depots show differential tendencies to increase in size as an individual becomes more obese. For example, more especially in human males, the paunch and subcutaneous fat in the thigh may be

greatly increased, whereas as the intramuscular fat in the calf hardly changes in quantity (Figure 1.14).

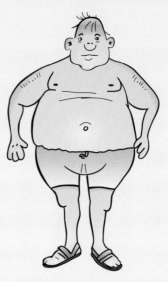

Figure 1.14 Fat depots in a human male.

Adipose tissue is usually seen as having a number of functions. You already know that the production of leptin by adipose tissue is a critical component of the homeostatic control of energy balance. In the longer term, adipose tissue may represent a significant energy store to be used in times of low energy availability. In humans, and other mammals, it is also known that release of fatty acids from adipose tissue is an important source of energy during intense or protracted exercise. Interestingly it turns out that there are substantial differences in the ability of different adipose tissue depots to release fatty acids at such times. Much of the release comes from subcutaneous fat rather than, for example, fat in the abdominal paunch. Raised levels of adrenalin in the blood stream together with release of noradrenalin from the sympathetic nerve endings within adipose tissue triggers this process.

It is also increasingly clear that adipose tissue plays a critical role in the homeostasis of fatty acid levels in other body tissues such as the muscles and the liver. This insight has come, in part, from the study of individuals who have abnormally low levels of adipose tissue, a condition known as congenital lipodystrophy. An example is the rare Berardinelli–Seip syndrome which results from a mutation in one of several genes coding for the enzymes critical to the synthesis of triacylglycerols from fatty acids.

● Why would an inability to synthesize triacylglycerols impair the ability to store fat in adipose tissue?

◐ In Book 1, Section 3.4 you read that triacylglycerols are the form in which fat is stored within adipose tissue. Triacylglycerols are synthesized from glycerol and the fatty acids that result from digestion of fats in the diet. A loss of the synthetic pathway for triacylglycerols prevents adipose tissue from storing fat, and the consequence during development is that very little adipose tissue is produced.

One result of congenital lipodystrophy is that high levels of fatty acids accumulate in both muscle and liver. Ironically, people with lipodystrophy share many physiological characteristics with those who are obese. In particular they develop insulin resistance and type 2 diabetes by early puberty. This occurs because the high levels of fatty acids in muscle and other internal organs disturb signalling initiated by the binding of insulin to the insulin receptor. Of course, another characteristic of those with lipodystrophy, but one that distinguishes them from obese individuals, is that they have very low circulating levels of the hormone leptin.

● What are the likely consequences of low leptin levels in these individuals and how might they be treated?

◐ The low levels of leptin will lead to enhanced appetite as a consequence of increased NPY and decreased α-MSH levels in the hypothalamus. The increased food intake will simply exacerbate the increased levels of fatty acids within muscle and liver. One potential treatment would be to administer leptin. Early indications (2004) are that this strategy may be successful.

A further function of one specialized form of adipose tissue is heat generation from metabolism of fat. Most adipose tissue has a white appearance, but one specialized form is light brown in appearance. The brown colouration arises from a high concentration of mitochondria within these adipocytes. The normal function of mitochondria is to produce ATP, which is used to provide the chemical energy necessary for the synthesis of complex molecules, such as protein, and many other processes vital to the maintenance and growth of cells (Book 1, Section 3.2.2). However, in the mitochondria within brown adipose tissue the usual production of chemical energy in the form of ATP can be *uncoupled* from the oxidative breakdown of fatty acids, sugars and amino acids shown in Figure 3.3 of Book 1. Since a basic law of thermodynamics states that energy cannot be lost, but only transformed from one form to another, the chemical energy that would have been stored in the ATP must appear somewhere else. In fact it is released from the cell in the form of heat. This uncoupling can be switched on by the release of noradrenalin from the sympathetic nerves that innervate brown adipose tissue. Heat generated by brown adipose tissue metabolism is of particular importance in infants who have a greater surface area to volume ratio than have adults, and also in the process of cold adaptation. At one time it was thought that the stimulation of heat generation by brown adipose tissue metabolism might produce a novel treatment of obesity in which, analogous to regulation of fluid balance by the kidney, energy balance could be achieved by increasing energy loss rather than by restricting energy intake. However, it remains unclear whether adult humans retain enough brown adipose tissue to make a real difference to total energy balance. In addition, it has not proved an easy matter to design drugs that act selectively at the noradrenergic receptors in adipose tissue without having unacceptable side effects elsewhere in the body.

In the same way, as a study described by Blundell et al. (2003) makes clear, exhortation to exercise may also not be very fruitful. In a four-week experiment, both normal and overweight women were prescribed the levels of exercise recommended by the World Health Organization (20 minutes aerobic activity 3–5 times a week). However, there was little effect on either energy expenditure or body weight in the participants, although the prescribed level of activity would have been predicted to lead to a loss of more than 1 kg providing energy intake did not change. The authors reported that their participants found even these moderate levels of activity hard to achieve and speculated that individuals who are already vulnerable to obesity in later life are unlikely to follow a prescribed exercise programme without considerable additional support. Nevertheless, epidemiological data (e.g. Sternfeld et al., 2004) do suggest that even mild exercise over a prolonged period is associated with a worthwhile reduction in the normal age-related increase in body weight observed in middle-aged women.

As you read in Book 1, Section 3.2.2, current drug treatments for obesity are limited, in part because of problems with side effects. One recent (2004) development, currently in late phase clinical trials, is a drug, known as rimonabant, which is an antagonist at the brain receptors for cannabinoid neurotransmitters. These are the same receptors that mediate the effects of tetrahydrocannabinol (THC), the most active component of marijuana ('grass' or 'hash') and they are found, amongst other places, in the ventral striatum (Figure 1.9). Interestingly, one side-effect of marijuana use, first reported more than 2000 years ago, is stimulation of appetite ('the munchies').

● What effect would you expect a cannabinoid antagonist to have on food intake?

● It should have the opposite effect to marijuana or THC and reduce food intake.

It may be that short term prescription of drugs similar to this, in combination with interventions that are aimed at longer term changes in an individual's diet and activity patterns, will provide more successful therapeutic options for the overweight and obese.

Summary of Section 1.3

1   Obesity is determined by a number of factors including environmental variables, such as the macronutrient content, energy density and fat content of available diets. Using whole room indirect calorimetry it has been found that humans are not good at recognizing the difference between low and high energy diets. Furthermore fat is less good at inducing satiety than are either carbohydrate or protein.

2   An evolutionary perspective offers an explanation for our inability to choose diets of appropriate energy density, and it is based on an assumption that we are adapted to survive in a very different environment to the one that currently prevails in developed countries.

3   Palatable foods appear to stimulate the mesolimbic dopamine system (a system also stimulated by sex and drugs such as cocaine). Feeding may be associated with increased release of dopamine in this system. Obese individuals have lower dopamine receptor availability in this system but it is not known whether this is cause or effect.

4 Increased weight with age might be a consequence of a reduced pattern of activity or a decrease in basal metabolic rate but, when measured in a longitudinal study, it might be attributable to cultural changes in eating habits.

5 Evidence that body weight has a heritable component comes from studies of adopted individuals and their biological and adoptive parents.

6 The thrifty genotype hypothesis has been proposed to explain the tendency for some specific groups to veer toward obesity when exposed to the energy-dense diets of the developed world.

7 A few cases of obesity are attributable to gene defects. These include an inability to produce leptin and faults in the production of human MC_4 receptors.

8 It is notoriously difficult to persuade overweight individuals to stick to a regime that involves taking exercise and reducing calorific intake. Feeding is a pleasurable experience, and hopefully a better understanding of its cellular basis will facilitate the development of drugs that will reduce the food reward and hence appetite.

1.4 Change

You now can see how genes and environment have, together, made you unique and also how this is a continuous and a continuing process. It is the continuing aspect that presents us with another of life's challenges. The processes of growth and development seem very positive up to the point where we achieve maturity. But why do we decline, both physiologically and psychologically, with advancing age? This, surely, is change we could do without!

As you studied the body systems, there were indications given of the way that each system changed with age. This next section summarizes some of the changes, particularly noting interactions between physiological processes and the way they affect psychological well-being. Although we will not discuss the biochemical and cellular bases of ageing, we will provide an evolutionary perspective.

1.4.1 The physiology of ageing

To judge from today's newspaper (2 January 2005) one aspect of ageing that concerns us is the appearance of skin. The paper has two articles on treatments that claim to reduce or remove wrinkles. Wrinkles are almost synonymous with ageing. This does seem to be a change that affects every one of us as we get older.

● Can you remember how wrinkles are formed (Book 1, Section 2.9.4)?

● In the dermis there are bundles of collagen fibres. Collagen is a fibre that has tremendous strength and elasticity, but the elasticity decreases gradually as we age and so skin loses its firmness and begins to sag or wrinkle.

In addition, the proportion of collagen in the skin increases and the water content of the connective tissue decreases with age. This increase in collagen and decrease in water content, coupled with the thinning of the fat layer just below the surface of the skin leads to the rather 'loose' and dry texture of ageing skin

(Figure 1.15). As far as we know at present, these changes are not reversible although many a fortune must have been made in persuading people that the application of creams containing collagen and 'moisturizers' would rejuvenate their tissues.

Figure 1.15 Photograph of a 90-year-old woman.

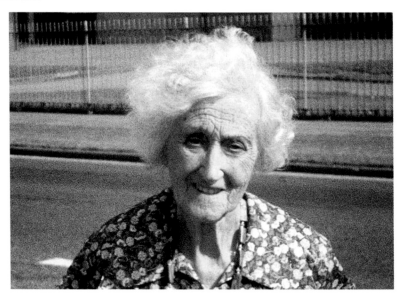

The appearance of an ageing skin has become associated with unattractiveness, especially by some women, and can therefore have harmful effects on their sense of well-being. In contrast, a 'glowing' tan is highly prized in some modern cultures. Ironically, prolonged sunbathing by light-skinned people increases the damage caused by ultraviolet radiation from the sun, the long-term effects of which are premature skin ageing, as well as increased susceptibility to skin cancer.

Decreased elasticity not only leads to wrinkles, but also to more global changes in facial features. For example, the soft areas below the cheek bones and jaw tend to droop. Another more global change in facial features associated with ageing occurs because cartilage continues to grow throughout life. As a consequence, the ears and nose, which are both supported by cartilage, become proportionately larger in relation to the other, bony structures of the skull. Psychological studies in which the participants are asked to estimate the age of individuals whose photographs have been manipulated to exaggerate or minimize each of these cues to age show that each of these factors is important in making age judgements.

Collagen is the most abundant protein in mammals so the fact that its structure alters with age has widespread effects. Its decreased elasticity is a consequence of cumulative cross-linking of collagen molecules that begins during youth. Cross-linking results from a spontaneous reaction between certain sugars (such as glucose and fructose) and part of an amino acid component of the polypeptide chain. This reaction is called glycation (Book 2, Section 3.7.2) and it is particularly prone to occur when glucose levels are high as in untreated diabetes. Glycation can affect any protein, but is likely to be especially important for long lasting proteins including collagen.

● Can you think of any other examples of age-related deterioration that might involve glycation of a protein?

● In Section 2.5.2 of Book 2, it was mentioned that cataracts are common in older people.

The proteins of the lens are called crystallins and are also subject to glycation. As they denature with age, they reform as cloudy deposits. But it is the decreased elasticity of collagen that probably has the most widespread potential for causing functional deterioration in body systems, from joints and skin to kidney, heart and lungs.

● How would the kidney and skin be functionally affected if their collagen content was more rigid?

● The filtration properties of the kidney would be adversely affected (Book 3, Section 1.3.1). Skin loses its elasticity and this may affect wound healing (Book 1, Section 2.10).

The question is, to what extent are these age-associated changes life threatening rather than merely inconvenient? One way of answering this question is to look at functional capabilities in body systems as they age. We can see in Figure 1.16 that there is a decline with age, for example note the decline in cardiac output (measured here as amount of blood pumped by the heart in one minute). Notice that the decline is represented as the function remaining expressed as a percentage of the function that was available at 30 years of age.

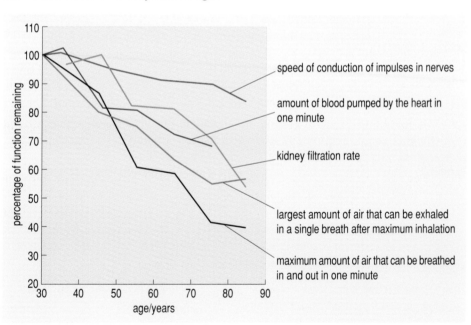

Figure 1.16 Decline in performance of some organs in humans with increasing age.

● Use Figure 1.16 to estimate the amount of blood pumped by the heart in 1 minute and the maximum amount of air that can be breathed in and out in 1 minute by a 70-year-old as a percentage of similar values for a 30-year old.

● The 70-year-old is pumping blood with about 70% of the efficiency of a 30-year-old, but the maximum amount of air that can be breathed in and out has been halved compared to that of the 30-year-old.

● Does this mean that the lungs are closer to the point where they will fail to meet the needs of the body than is the heart?

● Not necessarily. There are a number of points to consider, such as how much reserve capacity there was at 30 years of age. In other words, the average 30-year-old may well have a heart and lungs that have outputs that are way in excess of normal day-to-day needs.

Consider first the lungs. In Book 3, Section 3.2.2, the tidal volume (the amount of air normally breathed in and out) is shown to be only about one-eighth in men (about 13%) and one-fifth in women (20%) of the maximum intake possible in forced inspiration and about one-third (33%) of the amount possible in forced expiration. So, provided that the respiratory surfaces are functioning normally, a 50% drop in reserve capacity as seen by 70 years of age still leaves the lungs a long way from failing to provide an adequate service for most day-to-day activity (although the potential for athletic performance is much diminished!). In other words, the lungs have no problem in providing the tidal volume so far as we can judge from Figure 1.16. The question remains as to why there has been any loss at all.

● What suggestions can you make to account for the reduced ability to fill and empty the lungs in forced breathing?

● The lungs contain a lot of collagen fibres, and, as you know, this protein loses its elasticity with age. For the same reason there is less flexibility in the cartilage found in the ribs and sternum and this means that rib movements are restricted and hence forced breathing is less effective.

Turning now to the heart, Figure 1.16 shows the decline in cardiac output with age. You might recall that the resting output can double at times of anxiety or excitement (Book 3, Section 2.4.4; see also Table 1.2 below).

Table 1.2 Effect of various conditions on cardiac output. Approximate percentage changes are shown in parentheses.

Condition or factor	Effect
sleep	no change
moderate changes in environmental temperature	no change
anxiety and excitement	increase (50–100%)
eating	increase (30%)
exercise	increase (up to 70%)
high environmental temperature	increase
sitting or standing from lying position	decrease (20–30%)
rapid arrhythmia (heart beating irregularly)	decrease
heart disease	decrease

Even doubling the output does not take the heart's pumping capability anywhere near its limit, as it is estimated that the pumping capability is up to 400% above that normally required by the body.

● Figure 1.16 shows a drop of 30% by age 70. What reserve does this suggest?

● The fall of 30% in reserve capacity means that 70% remains:

$$400 \times \frac{70}{100} = \frac{28\,000}{100} = 280\%$$

So even by 70 years of age there is a reserve of 280%. Thus, even at times of excitement or anxiety, the aged heart should be able to maintain a sufficient cardiac output to meet the body's needs.

Thus, the drop in reserves with age, as indicated by Figure 1.16, does not suggest that the normal ageing processes push the body over that line from life to death. However, as we age we are often operating close to the limits of our reserves and are less able to respond effectively to challenges from the environment. For example, the skin, which is the largest organ in the body, is one of the places where temperature perception occurs. Temperature regulation is of fundamental importance in the maintenance of bodily function. Cold receptors are highly dependent on a good oxygen supply to function correctly. An age-associated deterioration in the blood supply to the skin may lead to a decline in function of the temperature receptors. This, coupled with alterations in the nerves controlling vasoconstriction and vasodilation, will also alter the way in which the body regulates temperature.

● Are there other aspects of the biology of ageing that could alter an older person's ability to regulate temperature satisfactorily?

● Muscular activity generates heat, but many old people have reduced mobility for a variety of reasons.

In very cold weather, the inability to regulate body temperature can lead to hypothermia which has resulted in a number of deaths in older people.

● What are the other, non-biological, factors that are responsible for an older person becoming hypothermic?

● Living in a cold damp house or flat with little or no heating, not being able to afford, or thinking that one cannot afford fuel, are likely to account for more deaths due to hypothermia than the age-associated changes in the ability to regulate body temperature. (Having someone else to light a fire or fill a hot water bottle if your mobility is restricted can make a world of difference. In other words, your social circumstances play a vital role in keeping warm.)

This awareness that the individual's experience of age and the healthiness of their later years is dependent on far more than their biology has been recognized by the UK government in formulating an action plan (in November, 2004) that fuel poverty will be eradicated by 2010 for elderly people. However, state intervention is only one part of the answer to the problem of coping with the challenges of ageing. The value of social support as a resource for maintaining health and well-being has long been recognized. In England, a classic study by

Brown and Harris (1978) emphasized the protective element in social support, and recent data show that higher levels of social support are associated with reduced levels of mortality and morbidity. There are two main theories to explain how social support affects health. One is that it directly and intrinsically enhances health and well-being. The other is that it acts as a buffer or cushions people against the effects of stressful experiences and so helps them to cope with stress. (See Chapter 3 for more on stress.)

What do we mean by the term 'social support' and who provides it? Social support simply means the support that people give and take within close social relationships. This usually includes family, friends and neighbours. It is informal, unlike the formal support that might be given by statutory workers such as social workers and care assistants. There are two aspects to social support. One is the emotional impact of love, affection and affirmation and the other is the practical help and advice that people get from their social relationships. This is important, not just in terms of the actual help, but for knowing that there is someone there to call on in an emergency.

The increased risk of chronic conditions which give rise to unpleasant symptoms, such as pain or disability, in older people, coupled with the increased likelihood of encountering bereavement (see Figure 1.17), accompanied frequently with a loss of income, all indicate that practical and emotional support in old age is vital. At the same time, the available pool of social support may, through death, marital break-up or geographical mobility, be dwindling. Nevertheless, the bulk of practical support given to older people is largely informal and comes from kin.

It used to be a frequent assertion that families in Britain neglected their elderly kin. This generated a great deal of research in the 1980s which showed that, on the contrary, families took on the bulk of the care of older people. Those older people who were without families or had outlived their children in some cases, were most at risk of both illness and death.

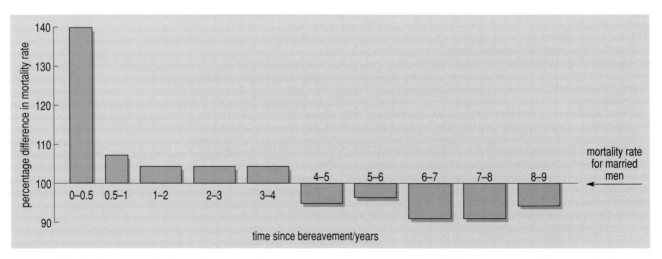

Figure 1.17 Mortality rate of widowers aged over 54 years as a percentage of the rate for married men of the same age. Note how the mortality rate of widowers in the first six months after the death of their spouse was 40% higher than the expected rate of deaths for married men of similar ages.

1.4.2 Evolutionary theory and ageing

The changes that occur as we grow and develop into mature adults are of clear functional value but the changes that occur subsequently do not benefit us as individuals. Why do we not keep our youthful looks and energy until the end?

When we make comparisons with other species we see that humans are extreme with regard to the proportion of individuals within the population who survive long enough to show clear signs of ageing. This is particularly true of affluent societies. It was pointed out earlier that we vary enormously from one to another, and this is particularly true in the particular signs of ageing that we display and in their order and onset. As some of these changes are unpleasant and debilitating, it seems reasonable to wonder why natural selection has not resulted in a greater proportion of the population being free from those age-related characteristics that disadvantage them.

● From your own perspective give some examples of age-related changes that are disadvantageous, and explain how they would disadvantage you. Would these examples have affected your ancestors too?

● Your list will reflect your current lifestyle in many ways and the items on your list will probably depend on your age. If you enjoy energetic sports such as squash or football, you might have cited loss of mobility preventing you from enjoying these sports and the associated social life. If your mobility is already somewhat reduced, you might be more concerned that reduced vision would prevent you from driving a car, or making use of public transport, and might hence result in a more isolated life.

If we speculated about our distant ancestors, we could imagine that both reduced vision and reduced mobility would affect their ability to hunt for or gather food.

Any individual who was less well equipped to compete for the resources essential for life would be at a disadvantage. The theory of natural selection predicts that those individuals, being less well adapted, would leave fewer surviving offspring. Over time, the proportion of the species that shares the adaptive characteristics rises.

● How then can these non-adaptive features persist? (*Hint*: Remember from Book 1, Section 1.4.2 that natural selection favours those characteristics that are both adaptive *and* are inherited by the organism's offspring.)

● One answer to this question is that the characteristic features of ageing are mostly 'beyond the reach' of natural selection because they appear well after reproduction has started and will have already been passed on to the offspring before they start to represent a disadvantage to the adult with the feature. Similarly, genes for longevity (which have certainly been identified in some species) will not increase in the population through the process of natural selection.

There are many different manifestations of ageing and if someone exhibits a characteristic that shortens their life and, more critically, results in their leaving fewer children than other people, then their biological fitness has been reduced. So natural selection would be operating in this example. But, in general, we don't die from age-related causes whilst we are still capable of producing fertile gametes, bearing children and caring for them.

1.4.3 Evolutionary theory and the menopause

This brings us to a second feature of our species. Human females lose the ability to ovulate, and therefore to bear children naturally at menopause, and this is usually long before they die. Various arguments have been advanced to explain the evolution of menopause, some of which can be easily countered. For example, having read the earlier parts of this chapter, you might suggest that there is some biological constraint that does not allow eggs to remain capable of completing meiosis for more than about 45 years. However, this seems unlikely since some other species of mammal continue to reproduce for much longer than humans. Female elephants are known to reproduce in their 70s and some species of whale reproduce in their 90s. On the other hand, many other mammalian species do show cessation of reproduction well before death when held in captivity in situations where predation, disease and other random causes of death are minimized.

Alternative approaches suggest that menopause may be adaptive in some way. Fundamental to these is the idea of the reproductive effort involved. For women, giving birth and feeding babies involves considerable physiological stress and the former can result in death. These factors are likely to be of particular importance in humans, since our bipedal gait restricts the size of the birth canal and human babies have relatively large heads (Kirkwood and Austad, 2000). The risks of birth, to both mother and infant, are likely to increase with the mother's age. By preventing further reproduction, menopause removes the associated risks.

● Why is this adaptive? In what way will it increase a women's biological fitness?

● The concept of biological fitness requires a maximization of the number of children that are raised to the point where they themselves can begin to reproduce.

Children are dependent upon their parents and particularly their mothers for food, warmth and protection for a long time. Remember too that reliable forms of birth control have become available only relatively recently. A woman who dies in childbirth leaves all her existing dependants at risk. If mothers continued having children throughout their lives, they would eventually undertake a birth that was so stressful that they would die, or be so severely weakened that they could not continue to care for their existing offspring. Thus, menopause may be adaptive because it favours the survival of existing children, but at the expense of potential future children.

Another argument in support of menopause as an adaptive characteristic that enhances biological fitness is that post-menopausal women have a valuable contribution to make to ensure that close relatives (kin) have successful pregnancies and that their babies are properly cared for. The initial evidence for this idea was gleaned from animal studies showing that in certain species the larger the extended family of care-givers, the higher is the rate of survival of infants born into it. The extended family includes relatives such as older brothers and sisters, cousins, aunts and uncles and grandparents (Figure 1.18).

In humans, recent evidence gathered from multi-generational lineages of farming families in both Finland and Canada during the 18th and 19th centuries (Lahdenpera et al., 2004) strongly support this hypothesis. A woman's first pregnancy was earlier if her own mother was still alive, and a child's probability of survival was significantly greater if his, or her, grandmother was still alive at their birth, especially if the grandmother was aged less than sixty. Overall, it was clear that a grandmother could enhance both the total number and survival of

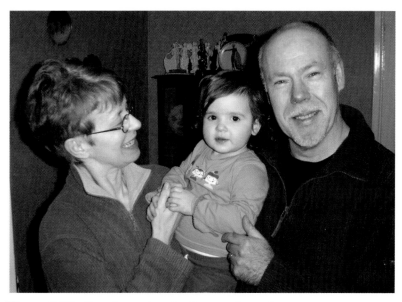

Figure 1.18 Grandparents enjoying a caring role.

her grandchildren and thus contribute to her biological fitness well after her own reproductive life was completed. Of course, the social structure was very different in these farming communities from that typical of present-day post-industrial society, but nevertheless grandparents today frequently have an important role in the physical, social and economic development of their grandchildren.

These two arguments suggesting that menopause is adaptive are not mutually exclusive; indeed it has been argued that it is only in humans that both factors are present, leading to the particularly obvious cessation of reproduction at menopause. Both hypotheses are based on an extension of the theory of natural selection called *kin selection*. According to either of the adaptive hypotheses for menopause that we have discussed, genes that cause a woman's reproductive activity to be switched off at a certain stage will be favoured by natural selection if, as a result of her post-reproductive behaviour, her progeny and those of other close relatives are more likely to survive. Her kin will tend to carry the same genes by descent, so the loss of reproductive potential by post-menopausal women is offset by her contribution to preserving the genes she shares with her kin. Thus the reproductive changes at menopause are believed to be adaptive, unlike other age-related changes, which are often likely to be beyond the control of natural selection.

● The emphasis in this section has been on the relationship between grandmothers and their grandchildren rather than grandfathers and their grandchildren. Why do you suppose this might be?

● Several possibilities may have occurred to you. It may be that, because of their previous experience of childrearing, grandmothers are especially able to provide help to their grandchildren. However, there is a quite different reason that may be significant. Arguments that involve kin selection require a clear specification of the genetic relationships between different individuals. It is easier to be certain about maternal than about paternal relationships and therefore to collect the necessary scientific data on reproductive success!

Summary of Section 1.4

1 As we age, there are a number of changes to our bodies, many of which are a consequence of changes to protein structure resulting from glycation.

2 Although there is a decline in functioning of the major organs with age, the body has substantial reserve capacity.

3 Social support is considered as a resource which can enhance health and well-being directly by providing love, affection and help; and indirectly by acting as a buffer between the individual and a stressful situation.

4 Menopause may be adaptive in preventing women from undertaking pregnancies throughout their lives. Without the menopause, the last-born children might not have their mothers around for long enough to rear them to the point of independence. A further benefit of menopause is that it may allow women a period in their life when they can offer their care-giver skills to close relatives, perhaps especially to their grandchildren.

1.5 Life's challenges

In this chapter we have examined the origin of genetic variability between individual humans. We have also seen that, at least in the case of obesity, this genetic variability interacts in a complex manner with the environment in which an individual develops. This is a conclusion that applies to many other domains of human physiology and behaviour. Only in rare cases will a mutation in a particular gene determine the timing and severity of a human disease. It is unlikely that variability in a single gene will ever be found to be responsible for the variability in a trait that lies within the range normally found within a population. So, there is no single gene 'for' obesity, or ageing, or aggression, or any other complex trait that you care to think of. However, that does not mean that variation in our genetic makeup does not contribute to the uniqueness that we develop as individual human beings. This should be kept in mind as you read the next two chapters.

In the last section of this chapter we examined some of the changes that arise as we progress through our life cycle. But there are other changes, imposed by our physiology, that we face every day. For example, we spend a considerable portion of each day sleeping and are so used to our regular sleep–wake cycle that we don't usually give it much thought. Indeed, many textbooks of human biology spend only a few pages describing the phenomenon. Yet, if you told an alien from another planet that individuals of the species *Homo sapiens* regularly and predictably went into a state where they were unaware of their surroundings and did not react to environmental stimuli, you might suddenly share their incredulity that intelligent beings could leave themselves so horribly vulnerable. And in today's 'time poor' world you might also wonder whether we really 'need' to engage in so much of this apparently useless activity. From your own experience you will very likely feel sure that you need to sleep, but that some other people seem to get by with very little sleep. What can human biology tell us about these issues? In the next chapter of this book we will find out more about sleep and the challenges that it presents.

We then consider another of life's challenges, often thought of as a very modern problem, that of stress. You will be aware that stress is a term that has constantly cropped up throughout this course, and you may already wonder whether the word has any distinct meaning and whether there is a science of stress. We intend that Chapter 3 will answer that question in a positive way!

In the final chapter of this book we return to the topic that began this chapter (completing another cycle!). The very special form of cell division known as meiosis provides the cellular basis for sexual reproduction and the genetic variability that it generates promotes evolution by natural selection. Chapter 4 will explore the biological processes that lead to production of sperm and eggs, to fertilization and pregnancy and finally to that hoped-for healthy baby.

Questions for Chapter 1

Question 1.1 (LOs 1.1 and 1.5)

Why, exactly, are characteristics, such as increased body weight, acquired during your lifetime unlikely to be directly inherited by your offspring?

Question 1.2 (LO 1.2 and 1.3)

Why are point mutations likely to have less severe effects than either frame shift mutations or the removal of one part of a chromosome to another chromosome?

Question 1.3 (LO 1.6)

Why has Ron increased in weight over the last few years?

Question 1.4 (LO 1.5)

An evolutionary perspective suggests that humans may not be well adapted to modern diets. Or, as George Bray (2004) put it, 'The genetic background may load the gun, but the environment pulls the trigger.'! A very different analogy sometimes used to describe the problem of trying to disentangle environmental and genetic influences is that it is like asking someone whether they use their right leg or their left leg for walking. Another analogy would be to say that it is like trying to identify the different contributions of eggs and flour to a tasty sponge cake. Comment on the advantages and disadvantages of these three analogies.

Question 1.5 (LOs 1.1, 1.2, 1.4 and 1.5)

Classify the following statements as true, partly true or false. Write a brief explanation, with examples, to justify your view.

(a) An individual's genotype, together with the environment in which he or she is currently living, provides the basis for his or her phenotype.

(b) Mutation is the process that leads to individual differences in genotype.

(c) *SRY* is a gene that suppresses ovarian development in the fetus.

(d) Each of the 64 possible codons in DNA codes for a different amino acid.

(e) Although parts of chromosomes might be lost after recombination, meiosis will always result in the same number of chromosomes in each gamete.

(f) Up to 40–60% of spontaneously aborted pregnancies have chromosome abnormalities, most of these being structural alterations.

References and Further Reading

References

Bindon, J. R. and Baker, P. T. (1997) Bergmann's rule and the thrifty genotype. *American Journal of Physical Anthropology*, **104**, 201–210.

Blundell, J. E., Stubbs, R. J., Hughes, D. A., Whybrow, S. and King, N. A. (2003) Cross talk between physical activity and appetite control: does physical activity stimulate appetite? *Proceedings of the Nutrition Society*, **62**, 651–661.

Bowlby, J. (1969) *Attachment and Loss: Attachment* (Vol 1). London: Hogarth Press.

Bray, G. A. (2004) The epidemic of obesity and changes in food intake: the Fluoride Hypothesis. *Physiology and Behaviour*, **82**, 115–121.

Brown, G. W. and Harris, T. O. (eds) (1978) *Social Origins of Depression: A Study of Psychiatric Disorder in Women*. London: Tavistock.

Farooqi, I. S., Keogh, J. M., Yeo, G. S.H., Lank, E. J., Cheetham, T. and O'Rahilly, S. (2003) Clinical spectrum of obesity and mutations in the melanocortin 4 receptor gene. *New England Journal of Medicine*, **348**, 1085–1095.

He, X. Z. and Baker, D. W. (2004) Changes in weight among a nationally representative cohort of adults aged 51 to 61, 1992 to 2000. *American Journal of Preventative Medicine*, **27**, 8–15.

Kirkwood, T. B. L. and Austad, S. N. (2000) Why do we age? *Nature*, **408**, 233–238.

Lahdenpera, M., Lummaa, V., Helle, S., Tremblay, M. and Russell, A. F. (2004) Fitness benefits of prolonged post-reproductive lifespan in women. *Nature*, **428**, 178–181.

McDonald's Corporation (2005) [online] Available from: www.mcdonalds.co.uk. (Accessed March 2005)

Ozanne, S. E. and Hales, C. N. (2002) Early programming of glucose-insulin metabolism. *Trends in Endocrinology and Metabolism*, **13**, 368–373.

Poppitt, S. D. and Prentice, A. M. (1996) Energy density and its role in the control of food intake: evidence from metabolic and community studies. *Appetite*, **26**, 153–174.

Prentice, A. M and Jebb, S. A. (2003) Fast foods, energy density and obesity: a possible mechanistic link. *Obesity Reviews*, **4**, 187–194.

Rolls, E. T (2004) Smell, taste, texture, and temperature. Multimodal representations in the brain, and their relevance to the control of appetite. *Nutrition Reviews*, **62** (Suppl. 11.1), 193–204.

Sternfeld, B., Wang, H., Quesenberry, C. P. Jr, Abrams, B., Everson-Rose, S. A., Greendale, G. A., Matthews, K. A., Torrens, J. I. and Sowers, M. (2004) Physical activity and changes in weight and waist circumference in midlife women: findings from the Study of Women's Health Across the Nation. *American Journal of Epidemiology*, **160**, 912–922.

Stunkard, A. J., Sorensen, T. I., Hanis, C., Teasdale, T. W., Chakraborty, R., Schull, W. J. and Schulsinger, F. (1986) An adoption study of human obesity. *New England Journal of Medicine*, **314**, 193–198.

Wang, G. J., Volkow, N. D., Logan, J., Pappas, N. R., Wong, C. T., Zhu, W., Netusll, N. and Fowler, J. S. (2001) Brain dopamine and obesity. *Lancet*, **357**, 354–357.

Williams, P. T. (1997) Evidence for the incompatibility of age-neutral overweight and age-neutral physical activity standards from runners. *American Journal of Clinical Nutrition*, **65**, 1391–1396.

Further Reading

Agarwal, A. K. and Garg, A. (2003). Congenital generalized lipodystrophy: significance of triglyceride biosynthetic pathways. *Trends in Endocrinology and Metabolism*, **14**, 214–221.

Horowitz, J. F. (2003) Fatty acid mobilization from adipose tissue during exercise. *Trends in Endocrinology and Metabolism*, **14**, 386–392.

Maynard Smith, J. (1998) *Evolutionary Genetics*, 2nd edn. Oxford: Oxford University Press.

Nuffield Council for Bioethics (2002) [online] *Genetics and Human Behaviour: the Ethical Context*. Available from: http://www.nuffieldbioethics.org/go/ourwork/behaviouralgenetics/introduction (Accessed March 2005)

O'Rahilly, S., Farooqi, I. S., Yeo, G. S. and Challis, B. G. (2003) Minireview: human obesity – lessons from monogenic disorders. *Endocrinology*, **144**, 3757–3764.

Pond, C. M. (1998) *The Fats of Life*. Cambridge: Cambridge University Press.

SLEEP

2.1 Introduction

Each of us, on average, spends about a third of our lives sleeping. Despite the fact that we devote so much of our time to it, most of us take sleep for granted and do not think about what sleep is or why we sleep. All of us, however, have been deprived of sleep at some time, or have had our sleep patterns disrupted, and know how lousy we feel as a result. Some people have medically recognized sleep disorders, such as insomnia, and for them sleep becomes a major preoccupation. Inadequate or unsatisfactory sleep is responsible for many accidents and is associated with poor health and with psychological problems (Section 2.6). The National Sleep Foundation of America recognizes sleep deprivation as a risk factor for developing a number of health conditions, such as type 2 diabetes, obesity and hypertension, whilst inadequate sleep has an immediate effect on mood, making sufferers prone to anger, anxiety or sadness. Clearly, we as individuals and society as a whole should derive considerable benefits from understanding sleep better than we do.

A major theme of the previous chapter that will emerge as you read this chapter is *variation*. While all humans share a vast number of characteristics that separate us, as a species, from chimpanzees or cats, each of us possesses unique characteristics that make us a distinct individual. In the context of sleep, some people habitually sleep a lot, others a little. Many people cannot wake up in the morning without the help of an alarm clock; many people wake up spontaneously.

● Looking at variation among people with respect to sleep is important for several reasons; suggest three of these reasons and their relevance to the study of sleep.

● (i) Describing variation is essential before we can determine the range of sleep patterns that are 'normal', and what is 'abnormal' or pathological. Individuals who sleep to excess, or who can't sleep at all, commonly experience problems in their work and social interactions and may seek medical treatment. What constitutes 'healthy' or 'unhealthy' patterns of sleep cannot be determined unless we understand variation between individuals.

(ii) Variation among individuals is a useful tool for studying a phenomenon of which we are rather ignorant, such as sleep. If we have a theory about the benefits of sleep, for example, an obvious way to test it is to compare people who sleep a lot with people who sleep a little, and to determine how other aspects of their lives, including their physiology, are different.

(iii) Variation based on genetic differences between individuals is an essential component of the theory of evolution by natural selection. A characteristic, such as how long we sleep, can only evolve if it, first, shows variation among individuals and, secondly, if that variation has some genetic basis. If sleep does have a genetic basis, this profoundly affects how we view variation in sleep among individuals, and how we might seek remedies for sleep abnormalities.

A second theme of this chapter is that, while scientists are gaining a greater understanding of sleep, our knowledge of it is much less than our ignorance. More importantly, the majority of the general public and those who determine our working lives are often not well informed about sleep. We could lead longer, healthier and more contented lives, and have fewer accidents, if society as a whole took more account of what is known about the biology of sleep.

This chapter reflects a common feature of the biological approach to humans in that it frequently talks about sleep in other animals. In this respect, it differs from the approach used in the earlier books of this course. This *comparative approach* is an important tool for understanding certain aspects of human biology, particularly behaviour. We can learn a great deal by studying animals that sleep more, or less than we do.

2.2 What is sleep?

The *Compact Oxford English Dictionary* (1996) gives the following definition of sleep: 'The condition of body and mind which normally recurs for several hours every night, in which the nervous system is inactive, the eyes closed, the postural muscles relaxed and consciousness practically suspended'. This definition may encapsulate what many people think sleep to be, but it is seriously wrong in several respects.

● In what ways would you take issue with this statement?

● Most importantly, the nervous system is definitely not inactive; if it were, our hearts would not continue to beat, etc. (Book 2, Section 1.8.2), nor would we have dreams. The muscles are not relaxed throughout sleep; most of us toss and turn in our sleep and some people go walking around the house (somnambulation). Whether or not consciousness is 'suspended' is a question that depends, as we will see, on what we mean by consciousness, an issue that we only lightly touched on in Book 2, Chapter 1.

One medical textbook defines sleep as 'a state of unconsciousness from which the person can be aroused by sensory or other stimuli' (Guyton and Hall, 1996). This definition separates sleep from other forms of unconsciousness such as that caused by a blow to the head. A person can be woken from sleep by external stimuli, such as the sound of an alarm clock. It is a common observation that parents of young infants can sleep through all kinds of noise but will awaken immediately if their baby makes the slightest sound. This suggests that we are rather selective about what stimuli will or won't wake us up, raising interesting questions about just how 'unconscious' or 'conscious' we actually are during sleep. Our perception is that our brain is inactive during sleep, but this clearly is not the case. As we will see later, the brain is as active during much of the time that we are asleep as it is when we are awake.

Many textbooks in the neurosciences avoid giving any kind of definition of sleep, clear evidence that it is a complicated phenomenon. Rather than seek a definition here, we will now look at various manifestations of sleep; this will introduce you to the very different aspects of sleep that are studied by scientists.

2.2.1 Sleep as behaviour

In humans, and in many other animals, sleep behaviour is typified by immobility, complete relaxation of the muscles, and a recumbent posture. None of these behavioural characteristics is absolute, however. Humans can fall asleep at a desk or driving a car. Humans and other animals change their posture frequently during sleep. Their eyes and, in cats, dogs and horses, their ears move about a great deal. Many animals sleep standing up; many birds do so standing on one leg. Humans, and many other animals, typically go to particular places to sleep, such as a bed, a burrow or a den. Common characteristics of such places are that they are comfortable, well insulated from the cold or shaded from the heat, and safe from external threats such as predators.

Another important behavioural aspect of sleep is that it occurs regularly at certain times of day. Humans, and most birds, sleep during the hours of darkness; badgers, foxes and owls sleep during the daylight hours. We will return to daily rhythms of sleep later in this chapter.

Finally, another behavioural manifestation of sleep is that it has a typical duration that is characteristic for a given species. Some species sleep a lot, others hardly at all. Some data for average sleep durations for a variety of species are shown in Table 2.1.

Table 2.1   Total sleep duration, per 24 h, for various species of mammal.

Hours	Species
20	two-toed sloth
19	armadillo, opossum, bat
16	lemur, tree-shrew
14	hamster, squirrel, mountain beaver
13	rat, cat, mouse, pig
12	chinchilla, spiny anteater
11	jaguar
10	hedgehog, chimp, rabbit, mole-rat, dolphin, dog
9	baboon, echidna
8	human, mole
7	guinea pig, cow
6	sheep, tapir, seal
5	horse, okapi, pilot whale
4	giraffe, elephant
0	shrew, Dall's porpoise

The figures presented in Table 2.1 need to be treated with caution. For most of the species listed, they represent average periods of inactivity, or 'apparent' sleep. To determine whether an animal is truly asleep requires attaching sensitive electrodes to their head to record brain activity. For obvious reasons, this cannot be done for animals leading normal lives. This dilemma illustrates why sleep is difficult to define. If sleep is defined according to physiological criteria, such as brain activity, we are limited to species and situations in which such investigations are possible. If sleep is defined in terms of behaviour, we have no way of knowing whether it is a similar phenomenon in humans and other animals.

2.2.2 The physiology of sleep

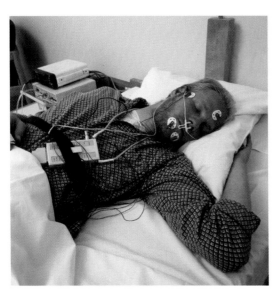

The state of the body during sleep can be studied by recording various aspects of a person's physiology while they are asleep. Sleep research thus involves finding ways of doing this that are as unobtrusive as possible. For example, body temperature can be recorded by means of a rectal thermometer, and frequent blood samples can be taken by means of a catheter, without the subject waking up. Such intrusions, combined with several electrodes attached to the head, are not everyone's idea of a good night's sleep, and research into sleep is hampered by the fact that it cannot be properly observed and recorded under normal conditions (Figure 2.1). This situation is improving, however, with the development of very small monitoring devices that people can carry around with them for several days.

Figure 2.1   A subject wired up for sleep recording in a sleep laboratory.

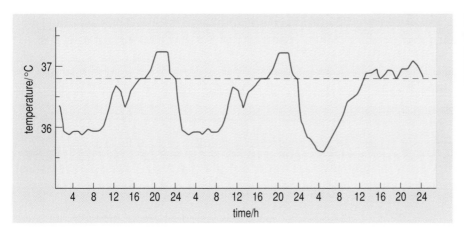

Figure 2.2 A plot of body temperature for one individual over the course of three days. The dotted line indicates what is referred to as 'normal' body temperature.

Body temperature is one of the easier variables to measure during sleep periods and Figure 2.2 shows body temperature measurements made over three days.

● What pattern does body temperature show over time?

● It shows a markedly rhythmical, or cyclic pattern with temperature reaching a peak each day from mid-evening to about midnight, then falling to a low point in the early hours of the morning.

Body temperature is showing a diurnal or **circadian rhythm** ('circadian' comes from the Latin, meaning 'about a day'). This rhythm is said to have a **period** of 24 hours, meaning that the time interval between any particular point in the cycle, such as its peak, is 24 hours.

Things are never simple in biology, and a major cause of complexity is individual variation. Figure 2.2 shows the temperature cycle of one person but we do not all show exactly the same pattern. In one study the temperature cycle of 101 young men and 71 young women was recorded over a six-day period (Baehr et al., 2000). The 172 participants were also asked to complete a variety of questionnaires, one of which categorized them as 'morning-types' (M-types), 'evening-types' (E-types) or as neither. M-types are typically alert in the morning and very sleepy towards bedtime; E-types are the reverse. M-types are often referred to as 'larks', E-types as 'owls'. The study found that the temperature cycle of M-types typically reached its lowest point at around 03:50 h, that of E-types at around 06:00 h. Participants categorized as 'neither' had a low temperature point at about 05:00 h. This study thus suggests that how our physiological state is synchronized with our sleep cycle can have a rather profound effect on how we function throughout the day.

● Look again at Figure 2.2. Was this recording taken from an E-type or an M-type person?

● An M-type; their temperature cycle reaches its lowest point at around 04:00 h.

Many other physiological processes show circadian rhythms, the most important of which in the context of sleep is the secretion of a hormone called **melatonin**, levels of which are much higher in the blood during the hours of darkness than they are during daylight.

Melatonin is secreted by a pea-sized organ, situated deep in the brain, called the **pineal gland**, or pineal body. (The philosopher René Descartes believed that, because the pineal gland is the only unpaired structure in the brain, it must be the location of the human soul.) Because melatonin is secreted into the blood, it travels to all parts of the body and so, potentially, can have some kind of effect on any part of the body.

● How is it that melatonin has effects on specific parts of the body?

● It will only affect those parts of the body that have specialized proteins called receptors that are responsive to it.

Melatonin receptors are known in only a few specific parts of the brain, the most important of which is a small, paired structure, the **suprachiasmatic nuclei (SCN)** that rests in the part of the brain known as the hypothalamus, close to the optic chiasma where the optic nerves cross – hence its name, *supra*, meaning above the optic *chiasma* (see Figure 2.3).

Light is detected by the specialized *melanopsin cells* in the retina of the eye, and signals are sent via the optic nerve to the SCN. From here, signals travel to various brain regions, including the pineal gland, which responds to these light-induced signals by switching off melatonin production.

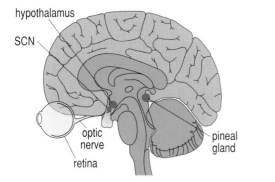

eye	the retina contains melanopsin cells that are sensitive to blue light
optic nerve	carries signals from the retina to the SCN in the brain
SCN: suprachiasmatic nuclei	a paired structure that controls the timing of physiological and behavioural rhythms, signals travel from here to the pineal gland
hypothalamus	controls body temperature, thirst, hunger and other physiological processes
pineal gland	pea-sized structure that secretes melatonin at night

Figure 2.3　Diagram of the human brain showing the position of structures involved in sleep, and their major functions.

Melatonin gets its name from the Greek word *melanos* meaning 'black'. It is secreted when the light intensity in the external environment is low, i.e. at night. Rather more is known about the way melatonin works in certain mammals than it does in humans. In particular, it plays a very important role in controlling reproduction in mammals that breed at specific times of year. Hamsters breed in the spring and are called a 'long-day species' because physiological and behavioural aspects of reproduction, such as an increase in gonad size, are stimulated by the steady increase in the light portion of the 24-hour day that occurs in spring. Sheep and red deer are 'short-day species'; they breed in the autumn and their reproductive activity is stimulated by the autumnal shortening of the light period. For both kinds of animal, melatonin provides the means by which the body detects the relative duration of light and dark periods. The period during which melatonin is secreted is decreasing in spring but is increasing in the autumn.

Humans are not seasonal breeders; they can reproduce at any time of year and women have an approximately 28-day reproductive cycle. Melatonin secretion patterns change significantly at puberty and at menopause, but whether correlations between these changes and reproductive status are functionally related is uncertain, particularly as, at both stages, secretion decreases. However, melatonin does appear to use the same biochemical processes to enable the body to detect the duration of light and dark periods, and thus to play a role in the control of sleep. Humans given melatonin in the evening become sleepy and fall asleep earlier than they otherwise would (Zhdanova et al., 1996). Melatonin is used by some people as a drug to offset sleep disruption caused by jet-lag. (It is not a drug available on prescription but it can be bought at health shops in many countries. However, because it interacts with growth hormone and the sex steroids in ways not fully understood, there is increasing concern about its 'over the counter' availability.) Melatonin is secreted in response to darkness and, as a consequence, humans secrete more in winter when nights are long than they do in summer. This may be related to forms of depression that affect some people in winter, ranging from the commonly experienced 'winter blues' to the more serious clinical condition **seasonal affective disorder (SAD)**, which has a very debilitating effect on a small proportion of the human population, especially at high latitudes. SAD is defined as a disorder in which the mood of the affected person changes according to the season of the year; typically, with the onset of winter, there is depression, general slowing of mind and body, excessive sleeping, and overeating.

● Why should SAD be more common at high latitudes?

● Because the nights are longer.

More importantly, perhaps, during winter months people are largely confined indoors where, although there is bright lighting, it may not be sufficient to be perceived by the brain as daylight, so that melatonin secretion is not fully suppressed during the day. Some patients with SAD can alleviate their symptoms by going out into daylight for one or two hours during winter. Others sit in front of extremely bright artificial lights that simulate natural daylight.

One leading researcher into SAD, Anna Wirtz-Justice, working in Switzerland (Wirtz-Justice, 1998), noticed that, as winter approaches, some of her patients behaved rather like short-day seasonal breeders such as hamsters. They increased their intake of energy-rich food and put on a lot of weight as a result. This suggests that, in at least some humans, the increased secretion of melatonin in winter may have physiological and behavioural effects. Hamsters are an example of a species that, in winter, goes into hibernation, a physiological state very different from sleep which involves a prolonged and dramatic drop in body temperature. Hibernation is an adaptive response to the hostile winter environment. Humans do not hibernate, but Anna Wirtz-Justice has suggested that the behaviour of some of her SAD patients may be a response to the onset of winter that could have been adaptive in the ancestral human environment (see Section 1.3.3).

While we are awake, there is a steady increase in the body of a chemical compound called adenosine (a compound containing nitrogen, sometimes used as drug to restore normal heart rhythm). This is broken down by physiological processes in the body during sleep. As it builds up during the day, it causes drowsiness, an effect that is blocked by two commonly used drugs, caffeine and nicotine (see *Brain Briefings*, 1998). Other physiological changes that occur during sleep are linked to specific types of sleep. These will be described in the next section, which looks at the complex way in which the nature of sleep varies during the night.

2.2.3 The neurophysiology of sleep

Our understanding of sleep, and of many other aspects of the working of the brain, was revolutionized, about 50 years ago, by the invention of the **electroencephalogram (EEG)** technique. **Encephalography** involves attaching electrodes to the skin of the head and recording minute variations in electrical activity, measured as voltage, that are generated by the brain. The electrodes are some distance from the brain and pick up variations in voltage that are the product, not of particular parts of the brain, but of the brain as a whole. The electrical activity is converted into a trace and this is commonly used in the diagnosis of epilepsy and brain tumours, conditions which cause characteristically altered EEG patterns (Book 2, Section 1.11.1).

Continuous EEG recordings taken while a person is asleep reveal a number of different patterns that represent different *phases* of sleep. Accounts of sleep vary in the number of these phases that they recognize, but all distinguish between two:

(i) **Rapid-eye-movement (REM) sleep**. Also known as active sleep, or paradoxical sleep. During REM, as its name implies, the eyes are moving about; the sleeper is dreaming.

(ii) **Non-rapid-eye-movement (NREM) sleep**. Also known as quiet sleep, deep sleep, synchronized sleep, or slow-wave sleep. NREM is often subdivided into four categories, called stages 1 to 4.

The EEG patterns typical of the five phases of sleep are shown in Figure 2.4.

You should not be concerned with exactly what the traces shown in Figure 2.4 represent; what is important is that the activity of the brain looks very different in the different phases of sleep. During the waking state, the EEG trace shows numerous, small 'spikes', within which there is no obvious pattern, indicating that the brain is very active. In stage 1 sleep, which corresponds to drowsiness, the trace shows fewer spikes, and there is an incipient rhythm developing. Stage 1 leads, through stages 2 and 3, to stage 4 sleep, in which a rhythm is very obvious.

● Look at Figure 2.4 and describe the period of these waves.

● They have a period of 0.5 to 2.0 seconds.

This rhythm consists of 'slow waves' also known as 'delta waves' and this phase of sleep is called 'slow-wave sleep'. During REM

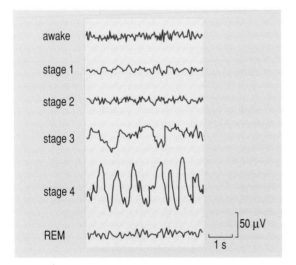

Figure 2.4 EEG patterns typical of a person while awake (top) and during the five phases of sleep.

sleep the pattern is very similar to that during wakefulness. (In our figure, stage 2 looks similar too.) The term 'paradoxical sleep' refers to the fact that, while the brain is as active as it is during wakefulness, the body is in a state of complete muscular relaxation that is quite unlike the wakeful state. The virtual paralysis of our muscles during REM sleep prevents us from acting out our dreams. (Interestingly, sleep-walking does not occur during REM sleep.)

During the course of a night, the brain cycles through the five phases of sleep a number of times, so that a sleeper has several bouts of each phase during the night (Figure 2.5). Note that bouts of deep sleep (phase 4) occur early in the night and that bouts of REM sleep get longer as the night progresses. It is the dreams that we are having in the final bout of REM sleep before we wake up that we remember. A person's behaviour on being wakened from sleep depends on the sleep phase they happen to be in at the time. People woken from deep sleep are generally very confused and have poor physical coordination; when woken from REM sleep, they are quickly awake, alert and able to function well.

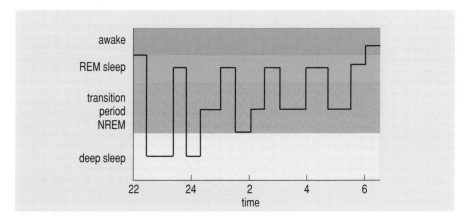

Figure 2.5   Cycles through sleep phases during the course of a night. 'Deep sleep' corresponds to stage 4 in Figure 2.4; 'transition period NREM' includes stages 1 to 3.

Modern methods such as PET (positron emission tomography) and fMRI (functional magnetic resonance imaging) scanning make it possible to see changes in the activity of different parts of the brain as they occur. These methods monitor, respectively, blood flow and oxygen consumption in the brain and thus reveal which parts of the brain are most active. Each phase of sleep has a characteristic pattern of brain activity, but the significance of this is not yet understood.

This brief account of what goes on in our bodies and our brains during sleep should have convinced you that sleep is a complex process. Before the invention of the EEG, sleep was regarded as an uninteresting phenomenon, one in which the brain is essentially 'switched off'. We now know that this is not the case; the brain is very active and there is considerable pattern and structure in this activity. We have to bear this complexity in mind later, when we ask a number of questions about sleep. In particular, when we ask a question such as 'what is the function of sleep?' we should clearly consider whether different phases of sleep might have separate and distinct functions.

2.3 Sleep and the biological clock

Humans and other animals could organize their sleep and other routine activities during the course of the 24-hour day-night cycle by responding directly to external stimuli; they could, for example, go to sleep when it gets dark and wake up when it gets light. If we did this, people living at high latitudes (e.g. in the UK) would find that we slept a lot in the winter and less in the summer. In general, living organisms do not respond directly to environmental time cues; instead, they respond directly to internal signals from a biological clock, which in turn can be influenced by external stimuli. This is a very basic feature of living organisms, occurring not only in animals, but also in plants and bacteria: in plants it controls leaf movements and the opening and closing of flowers; in bacteria, it controls activity according to the time of day.

To establish that an organism has a biological clock, and is not responding to cyclical changes in its environment, it is necessary to carry out a particular kind of experiment, called a **free-running** experiment, in which the organism is isolated from such changes. Under these conditions, organisms show a characteristic change in their behaviour and physiological processes. Figure 2.6 shows the activity of a cockroach, a nocturnally active animal, in a free-running experiment.

● Describe what happens to the cockroach's activity when the light is turned off.

● It becomes active.

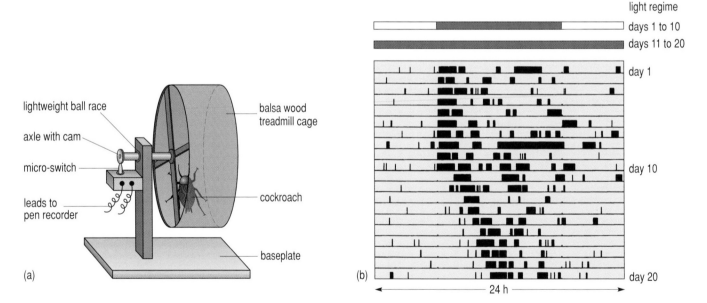

Figure 2.6   Cockroach behaviour under free-running conditions. (a) Apparatus for recording cockroach activity. The wheel rotates as the cockroach runs or walks, triggering a micro-switch connected to a pen-recorder. Food and water are supplied through a hole on the right-hand side of the wheel. (b) Activity record for a cockroach kept for 20 days in a running wheel. The lighting regime was 12 hours light alternating with 12 hours dark on days 1 to 10, switching to continuous darkness on days 11 to 20. Activity is shown as upward deflections of the trace, which become solid blocks when the cockroach is very active.

- What happens to the activity period of a cockroach when it is in continuous darkness?

- It shifts slightly each day so that, by day 20, it begins several hours later than it did on day 11.

Despite the difficulties encountered in setting up experimental protocols for humans, some similar experiments have been carried out on human volunteers. Participants are confined for many days in underground bunkers, where they have no access to clocks, or any other cues to the true time of day. They can eat, sleep, switch the lights on and off, etc. when they choose. Typically, humans do what cockroaches do and show a gradual delay, of about a hour, in their activities from day to day. As a result, participants kept like this for a month have lived through one less day/night cycle than people leading normal lives.

This typical pattern of gradually shifting activity under free-running conditions tells us something very important about the biological clock: it is not very accurate. You will recall that the term *circadian* rhythm means 'about a day', and this reflects the inaccuracy of the biological clock. In most people the natural period of their clock is around 24.5 to 25 hours, but a small proportion of the human population has a clock with a period just under 24 hours.

- How might this relate to the fact that some people are categorized as 'larks', others as 'owls'?

- 'Larks' appear to be people whose biological clock has a period just under or very close to 24 hours; they spontaneously wake up just before or just when they need to. 'Owls' have a clock with a period of more than 24 hours and tend to oversleep if they do not use an alarm clock.

'Larks' and 'owls' are recognized, in the jargon of sleep research, as distinct 'chronotypes' (from the Greek *chronos*, meaning 'time'). Comparisons between morning and evening chronotypes have revealed a number of differences between the two (Taillard et al., 2003). For example, the diurnal rhythm of body temperature peaks about two hours later in evening types than in morning types, and the build-up of subjective sleepiness is much slower in evening types. Such data support the hypothesis that individual differences in sleep patterns are linked to variations in the biological clock.

The biological clock is thus like a mechanical clock that keeps time rather poorly. Just as such a clock has to be corrected every day, so the biological clock is reset each day by a variety of environmental stimuli, such as daylight. In humans, social stimuli are very important regulators of the biological clock; we tend to adjust our behaviour to do what other people around us are doing. How our habits affect the behaviour of the molecular apparatus governing the internal clock is not known but schedules of physical activity to overcome the effects of say, changing shift work patterns or jet lag, may gradually reset the desynchronized clock.

Evidence for the existence of a biological clock also comes from the experience of jet lag. If we travel westwards through 90° of longitude, a quarter of the way around the world, we find on arrival that our biological clock is six hours out of synchrony with local time. As a result, we want to go to sleep when everyone

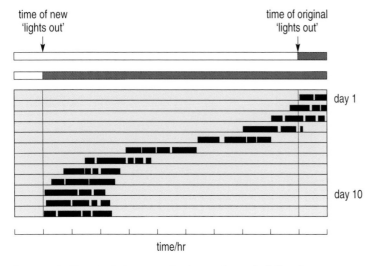

Figure 2.7 Activity record of a cockroach following a large change in the light/dark cycle. After day 1, the cycle was changed so that 'lights out' occurred 9 hours earlier.

around us is awake. Figure 2.7 shows the result of an experiment that simulates jet-lag in a cockroach; in this experiment, the light/dark cycle experienced by the cockroach was shifted abruptly by nine hours.

● How long did it take for the cockroach to resume its normal pattern of behaviour, such that it became most active just after lights-out?

● Nine days.

As for cockroaches, it takes several days for humans to recover from the effects of time-shifts caused by jet-lag. Many studies of human performance in a variety of manual and mental tasks show impairment due to jet-lag, and that recovery of normal function requires about one day for each hour of induced time-shift. The relationship between jet-lag, other kinds of time-shift and sleep patterns will be discussed further later in this chapter.

A great deal of research has been carried out, particularly on mammals such as rats and hamsters, to determine the location of the biological clock, and it is clear that the suprachiasmatic nucleus (SCN) plays a major role in time-keeping (see Figure 2.3). The SCN receives information about light levels in the external world, via the optic nerve, from special cells, called melanopsin cells, in the retina of the eye. This pathway appears to be quite separate from the visual pathways in the optic nerve that originate from the rods and cones found in the retina (Book 2, Section 2.3).

Summary of Sections 2.1–2.3

1 Sleep is a complex phenomenon, characterized by distinctive behaviour, physiological changes and neurological activity.

2 There is much variation among species in the number of hours per day spent in sleep.

3 In humans, there is variation in the duration of sleep and in the preferred timing of sleep.

4 EEG recordings reveal two major kinds of sleep, REM and non-REM sleep. Both occur in bouts during the night, with non-REM occurring mostly early in sleep, REM more towards the end.

5 The timing and duration of sleep are largely controlled by a biological clock in the brain, located in the SCN.

6 Melatonin, a hormone secreted by the pineal gland and implicated in the control of seasonal breeding and hibernation in animals, is thought to play a role in the control of sleep in humans.

2.4 Sleep and the life cycle

During the course of our lives, our patterns of sleep change in a variety of ways. Infants sleep an average of 16 hours per day, teenagers nine hours, and adults between five and ten hours. The sleep of older people tends to be more interrupted during the night by periods of wakefulness. A detailed study of sleep patterns of 989 adults in Switzerland looked at a number of factors that influence sleep duration, including season and gender (Wirz-Justice et al., 1991). (Women sleep for slightly longer than men and both sexes sleep for longer in winter.) This study revealed that, with advancing age, people sleep for a shorter time at night and are more likely to take a nap during the day. In the 20–30 age group, 12.6% of participants took naps, whereas 66.7% did so in the 80–90 age group.

A comparison of young adults (aged 18–32) and older adults (60–75), who were healthy and reported no sleep problems, revealed that younger adults generally nap in the afternoon, whereas older people nap in the evening, especially within two hours of bedtime (Yoon et al., 2003). Napping was associated with reduced nocturnal sleep time in older adults, but not in the younger group. This suggests that, if you are in the older age group and want a good night's sleep, it is best not to nap close to bedtime.

Sleeping during the day shows much cultural variation; people in southern European countries typically take a siesta, whereas people in more northerly latitudes, such as Britain, generally do not. This could be a direct response to very high daytime temperatures in southern Europe in summer, but it could also suggest that our patterns of sleep may, to some extent, be learned during early life.

In addition to changes in overall sleep duration, very interesting changes take place during our lives in the relative proportions of the different types of sleep during the night (Figure 2.8).

● What proportion of the sleep period consists of REM sleep in newborn infants?

● In newborn infants, 50% of the 16 hours spent in sleep consists of REM sleep.

● How does this proportion change with increasing age?

● It decreases. By 10 years of age and onwards, the proportion of REM sleep has declined to approximately 20%.

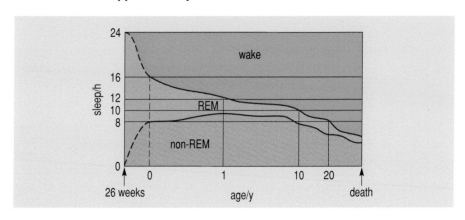

Figure 2.8 The proportions of a 24-hour day that are devoted to being awake, REM sleep, and non-REM sleep over the course of a human lifetime.

Figure 2.9 Changes with age in the proportion of total sleep consisting of REM sleep in three mammals.

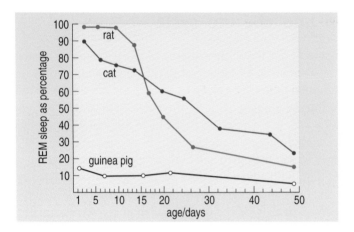

This effect is also apparent in studies of a number of other mammal species (Figure 2.9).

A remarkable result from studies of the development of sleep is that unborn infants spend 100% of their time in REM sleep (Figure 2.8). For obvious reasons, this phenomenon is difficult to study, but EEG recordings taken from premature babies show that, at 26 weeks gestational age, infants spend most of their time in REM sleep. Of the time spent in non-REM sleep, children show a higher proportion in slow-wave (stage 4) sleep than adults (Gaudreau et al., 2001).

Recently, doubts have been cast on the presumption that REM sleep is actually present in very young mammals, including humans. New-born mammals spend as much as 90% of their time in a sleep state characterized by frequent twitches, eye movements and irregular breathing. It is suggested that this is not actually REM sleep but is the result of irregular, spontaneous nervous activity which, with increasing age, becomes organized into the distinct states of REM and non-REM sleep. Thus, infant sleep may be a disorganized precursor to adult sleep.

Thinking about the development of sleep during life inevitably raises the question of whether it has some genetic basis. It could be that our sleep patterns are wholly determined by our genes, or it may be that our genes are irrelevant and that our sleep patterns are entirely determined by factors operating after conception. It is possible that we sleep for, say, eight hours, or are 'morning types' because we 'learned' these patterns in the womb from our mother.

Investigation of the possible genetic basis of sleep is in its infancy, but the following observations suggest that there may be some genetic component to our sleep patterns.

(i) Insomnia tends to run in families. This is consistent with there being a genetic component to sleep, but is not conclusive; insomnia could be passed on by social factors (Bastien and Morin, 2000). For example, *fatal familial insomnia* is a transmissible disease. (It is also an inherited disorder.)

(ii) No less than five separate genes have been shown to influence the biological clock in the fruit fly (*Drosophila*) and are also present in humans.

(iii) A human sleep disorder called *familial advanced sleep phase syndrome* (*FASPS*), so called because it runs in families, is strongly suspected of being caused by a mutant form of one of the clock genes that we share with *Drosophila*. People with FASPS have a circadian rhythm of sleep, temperature and melatonin secretion with a period of about 20 hours; they wake up spontaneously very early in the morning and have great difficulty staying awake in the evening.

2.4.1 Naps and micro-sleeps

While sleep is generally regarded as a night time activity in humans, most of us have short periods of sleep during the day. These range from a premeditated nap or siesta after lunch to 'micro-sleeps' that are so short that we are often not aware of them. In this section, we look briefly at deliberate napping as a strategy to make life better and at unintentional micro-sleeps that can have fatal consequences. A nap has no precise definition but usually refers to an intentional daytime sleep episode lasting from a few minutes to a few hours. Anything shorter than five minutes is called a micro-sleep.

> 'Napping works. It makes you sharper, smarter, happier and more energetic. It is safe, costs nothing and you need no special equipment or drugs to do it. And it feels good. Besides being a valuable skill, napping is one of the great, neglected pleasures of life.'
>
> (Martin, 2002)

A strong advocate of napping, the behavioural scientist Paul Martin considers an afternoon nap to be a natural expression of human biology, reflecting changes in our physiology, and a decline in alertness, that occurs in the afternoon. There is a substantial amount of research (e.g. Mednick et al., 2003) showing that an afternoon nap improves alertness, mood and performance on a variety of cognitive tasks, even if it lasts only 10 minutes, though 20 minutes is better. In recognition of the beneficial effects of naps, they are often referred to as 'power naps'. Martin distinguishes three types of nap, depending on their purpose:

(i)   prophylactic naps, taken in anticipation of sleep deprivation, a late night or a long journey.

(ii) relief naps, taken in compensation for lost sleep.

(iii) pleasure naps, taken because they feel good.

By contrast, micro-sleeps are not premeditated; people frequently fall asleep briefly without being aware that they have done so, unless it is for more than a few minutes. Research into daytime sleep has investigated the awareness of participants woken up after varying intervals. After one minute of sleep, only 15% of participants were aware that they had been asleep; after five minutes, only 35% were aware. Falling asleep without being aware of it can be a very serious matter, as we shall see in Section 2.5.

Summary of Section 2.4

1   Patterns of sleep change with age, people sleeping less at night as they get older, but tending to take naps during the day.

2   The proportion of sleep that consists of REM sleep declines with age.

3   There is evidence that some aspects of individual variation in sleep have a genetic basis.

4   Napping serves, in many people, to augment night time sleep and to improve performance and well-being.

5   Very short sleeps, or micro-sleeps, may occur frequently but are largely unnoticed.

2.5 The function of sleep

Before we consider the possible function of sleep, we have to digress briefly to discuss what we mean by the word 'function'. In everyday speech, the 'function' of a spade is to move soil. In evolutionary biology, however, the word means something much more precise, specific and complicated. An alternative expression that is often used in biology is 'survival value', but this does not fully capture what biologists mean by 'function'.

The function of a particular pattern of behaviour, such as sleep, is a precise measure of the contribution that that behaviour makes to an individual's fitness.

● What does the term 'fitness' mean to a biologist?

● The fitness of an individual is measured as its lifetime reproductive success relative to other members of the same species (Book 1, Section 1.4.2 and Section 1.3.3 of this book).

Expressed loosely, this means how sleep enhances an individual's survival and reproduction. However, biologists nowadays seek to measure the fitness of individuals very precisely, an undertaking that requires monitoring their survival, the number of their offspring, and the reproductive success of those offspring and of other close relatives. All this has to be done under natural conditions since laboratory studies do not help us to measure fitness. To give an example, to determine the fitness of individual red deer living on the Scottish island of Rhum with reasonable accuracy has taken a group of research biologists about 30 years of continuous study.

In practice, biologists seeking to determine the function of a behaviour pattern have to settle for assessing some consequence of that behaviour which it is reasonable to assume makes a contribution to fitness. There are three ways to approach the study of function.

1   *Looking at individual variation.* Some individuals sleep a lot, others a little. If sleep is beneficial we might expect the benefits to be more apparent in individuals that sleep a lot, less in those that sleep little. This is an approach that seeks *correlations* between sleep and other aspects of biology. There appear to have been few studies of human sleep that have used this approach. One that has sought evidence that REM sleep is important in memory formation, but found no evidence that people who have a lot of REM sleep have better memories (Siegel, 2001). Nonetheless, from what you have already read about sleep, there are some tantalizing clues. Sleep duration is related to age, for example, suggesting that it is more important when we are young. More specifically, REM sleep is more prominent in young people and other young animals.

2 *Experimental manipulation.* The objective in this approach is to experimentally decrease, or increase, the amount of sleep that individuals have and to see how this affects other aspects of their biology. Sleep deprivation experiments involve preventing participants, including non-human animals, from falling asleep; the results they yield are rather dramatic. Chronically sleep-deprived rats soon lost their ability to regulate their body temperature, they increased their feeding rate but nonetheless lost weight, they became very susceptible to infection, and died within three weeks. (Note: experiments like this were done many years ago; the change in ethical attitudes to animal experimentation means that such extreme experiments would not be allowed today.)

Sleep deprivation experiments with human participants reveal that quite small amounts of sleep deprivation lead to reduced performance on a variety of mental and physical performance tests. These provide the basis for the strict rules that govern the work and rest schedules in jobs where operator alertness is crucial, e.g. airline pilots, truck drivers, etc. A lot of research has focussed on the effect of sleep deprivation on memory formation. Participants trained on a variety of manual and mental tasks retain learned skills much better if they have normal amounts of sleep but, as we will see later, the interpretation of this effect is controversial. Other studies show, not surprisingly, that sleep deprivation impairs performance in exams. Overwhelmingly, studies show that it is deprivation of non-REM (NREM) sleep that does the damage. Adults deprived of REM sleep do not appear to perform less well in physical or mental tasks.

3 *The comparative method.* The aim of this approach is to gather data from a large number of different species and to see if variation in their sleep patterns correlates with other aspects of their life styles. You will recall from Table 2.1 that there is enormous variation among species in their average daily sleep duration, from 20 hours per day in the sloth, to none at all in some species of shrew. There is little that we can conclude about the function of sleep from these data, but animal studies do supply us with some important clues when we look at different components of sleep.

A comparative study of 69 mammalian species looked at the relative amounts of quiet (NREM) sleep and active (REM) sleep. Across these species, time spent in quiet sleep is negatively correlated with body size and with metabolic activity, meaning that larger and more active mammals engage in less quiet sleep than smaller and less-active species. The time spent in active sleep shows no relationship with either body size or metabolism, but is related to an aspect of life history.

Some animals are described as **precocial**, meaning that they are born at an advanced stage of development. They are born with open eyes, they can move about independently soon after birth and they require relatively little care from their parents; horses and cows are precocial mammals. In contrast, **altricial** species produce young that are blind at birth, often naked, unable to move about, and very dependent on parental care; cats are altricial mammals. You should not regard precocial and altricial as clear-cut, distinct categories. Rather, there is a continuum across species with more precocial species at one end, more altricial species at the other.

In the mammal study, time in active sleep was found to be greater in altricial than in precocial species, especially when they are young. This effect is apparent in Figure 2.9; the guinea pig is a more precocial species than the rat or the cat.

● Why do you think active sleep might be greater in altricial species compared with precocial ones?

● Active sleep could be important for brain development.

Precocial species have completed much of their brain development by the time they are born and this may be why they need less active sleep after birth. This fits rather well with the fact that, in humans, infants devote much more time than adults to REM sleep (Figure 2.8). Indeed, sleep disturbances are a significant factor in neurodevelopmental disorders affecting children. (Stores and Wiggs, 2001). This adds further support to the earlier suggestion (Section 2.4) that the REM sleep of adults is not the same activity as the supposed REM sleep of young mammals.

2.5.1 Theories about the function of sleep

The oldest and most widely held theory about the function of sleep is that it is a restorative or recuperative process. Our own personal experience tells us that sleep makes us more alert and better able to meet the demands of the daily grind. Personal experience and experiments on humans and other animals clearly show that sleep deprivation adversely affects physical and mental *performance* (there is no physiological impairment of the muscle tissue itself). We will return to this theory shortly, but first note that the comparative data shown in Table 2.1 raise some awkward questions about this theory. Shrews are very active, busy little creatures; how do they survive with no sleep at all? Sloths are slow-moving animals when they're awake; do they really do so much in four hours that they need 20 hours to recover?

Such questions have lead to the **ecological theory of sleep**. This explains sleep as an adaptation to two aspects of animals' lives. First, most animals do not need to be continuously active to find sufficient food, mate, and complete all the other activities that they do in their daily lives; they have 'spare time'. This could explain why carnivores (e.g. cats) that eat large meals of highly nutritious food, and therefore need only occasional meals, generally sleep more than herbivores (e.g. cow, giraffe) which eat food of low nutritional content and so have to feed for a large proportion of the day. Second, most animals are adapted, particularly with respect to their senses, for being active either in daylight or at night. Shrews and moles spend most of their time underground where it is permanently dark, but most monkeys, and humans, have poor nocturnal vision and are thus ineffective, during the night, at finding food, avoiding obstacles and seeing a predator before it sees them. The ecological theory of sleep is thus based on the idea that, for most animals, there are times in the day when the optimal thing to do is to keep out of harm's way.

Given that an animal is going to be inactive for a while, it makes good sense that it adopts a physiological state that minimizes its energetic needs and maximizes its safety. The reduction in body temperature that is characteristic of sleep reduces its energetic requirements; immobility makes it less conspicuous to predators.

The ecological and the restorative theories of sleep are not opposing, or alternative theories, but are fully compatible with one another. Once a species has evolved a daily period of sleep it obviously makes sense to use that time to recuperate. We must assume, however, that animals like shrews that do not sleep nonetheless need to restore themselves and have evolved some other way of doing so.

We have, so far, been rather vague about exactly what 'restoration' and 'recuperation' might mean in the context of sleep. Several hypotheses have been proposed for the recuperative role of sleep, none of which is mutually exclusive.

1   First, sleep has some role in maintaining 'homeostatic equilibrium'.

A study showed that a sleep deficit of 3–4 hours per night for a week affects the ability of the body to process carbohydrates, manage stress, and maintain a proper balance of hormones (Spiegel et al., 1999). During sleep, several hormones are secreted that affect growth, regulate energy and affect metabolic and endocrine functions. Growth hormone is secreted during sleep and this is of particular importance for childhood growth, and in regulating muscle mass in adults.

● In relation to stress and carbohydrate processing which hormone shows a diurnal rhythm?

● Cortisol. Figure 3.15 in Book 2 showed a lower level of secretion of corticosteroids through the night with levels rising a few hours before waking.

The sleep cycle also affects the secretion of the hormone leptin, which has a direct influence on appetite and weight.

2   Second, sleep conserves energy.

3   Third, sleep facilitates tissue repair.

Active cells become damaged and sleep allows them to be repaired. Evidence in support of this is provided by the fact that the production of proteins, the 'building blocks' of cells, increases in the brain at night.

4   A fourth, and most controversial, function that has been suggested for sleep, especially REM sleep, is that it consolidates memory and improves learning.

Dreaming is seen as an important part of this process. A number of studies using humans and other animals have shown that new tasks are learned less well if the first experience of them is followed by sleep deprivation. This could, however, be the result of other physiological effects caused by sleep loss, rather than of a specific effect on memory formation. That the role of sleep in memory formation is controversial is shown by three major reviews, published side by side in the leading journal *Science* in 2001 (see Further Reading; *Science*, 2001). These concluded that: '… evidence for the influence of sleep discharge patterns on memory traces remains fragmentary'; 'evidence supports a role for sleep in consolidation of an array of learning and memory tasks'; 'although sleep is clearly important for optimum acquisition and performance of learned tasks, a major role in memory consolidation is unproven'. Scientists working at the frontiers of science rarely agree with one another!

More direct evidence that sleep is involved in the consolidation of complex cognitive processes comes from fMRI studies that reveal high activity in the cingulate prefrontal arc areas of the brain during sleep. These are the same regions that are especially active in individuals who are awake and who are carrying out a diverse array of cognitive tasks.

5   Finally, it has been suggested that sleep plays a role in the body's immune defences against infection.

The immune response is an extremely complicated system, involving the production of a diverse array of chemical compounds and of several different types of cells (Book 3, Chapter 4). Several of these compounds, e.g. adenosine, show an increase in concentration in the blood during sleep, and injection of some of them into the blood induces sleep (Krueger et al., 1999). Certain cytokines produced by the immune system to combat infection have sleep-inducing properties. For example blocking interleukin-1 (first mentioned in Book 1, Section 2.12) and tumour necrosis factor-a alters the regulation of sleep in the normal brain. (Vitkovic and Bockaert, 2000). You may have noticed that humans and other animals tend to sleep more when they are suffering from an infection. The interaction between the immune system and the nervous system, variously referred to as 'psychoneuroimmunology' or 'immunopsychology' is an area within the neurosciences that is increasing in importance.

We have seen that sleep is a complex phenomenon, with several distinct phases. This raises the possibility that the different phases serve different functions. The adverse effects that are observed following deprivation of NREM sleep suggest that this is the phase that allows recuperation and restoration to occur. Being deprived of REM sleep has negligible adverse effect. The higher incidence, in humans and animals, of REM sleep during early life, combined with the higher levels of REM sleep seen in the young of altricial species, suggests that it plays a role in brain development. From early times many cultures have focussed attention on the possible functions of dreaming. The finding that adults only dream during the REM phase of sleep has not diminished scientific interest in this phenomenon.

2.5.2 The evolution of sleep

Virtually all animals, and plants, are more active at some times of day than at others, simply because their environment changes on a cyclical, daily basis. Only organisms that live deep underground or in the depths of the sea live in an environment that does not change during the course of the day. Most animals become inactive and hide away during some part of the day or night to avoid heat, cold or darkness. Some coral reef fish, for example, lie on the sea-bed at night and, interestingly, lose their bright colours. Behaviour that has much in common with human sleep is thus nearly universal. Sleep in humans, however, is a complex physiological state and it is very unlikely that it is similar across all animals.

An interesting form of sleep occurs in dolphins, mammals which cannot rest because they have to swim continuously. They sleep while swimming, and EEG recordings show that only one side of the brain sleeps at a time. One side sleeps for about two hours, then both sides are awake for one hour, then the other side sleeps for two hours, and so on, for about 12 hours per night (Figure 2.10).

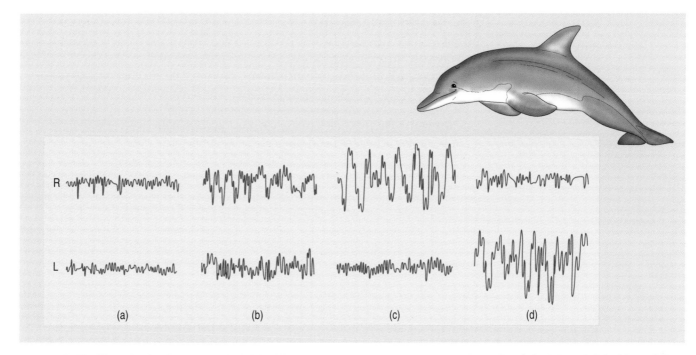

Figure 2.10 Sleep in the bottlenose dolphin. These EEG recordings were made from the right (R) and (L) sides of the brain. (a) High-frequency activity on both sides during wakefulness. (b) Slow-wave sleep on the right side. (c) Slow-wave sleep on the right side, high-frequency activity on the left. (d) As in (c), but with the sides of the brain reversed.

While the duration of sleep, and the temporal patterning of its different phases varies a lot between species, its underlying physiology is similar among those mammals that have been studied, suggesting that it was probably present in the earliest ancestors of mammals. Birds sleep for long periods, usually adopting a distinctive posture, such as tucking the beak under a wing; some parrots sleep hanging upside-down like bats. Birds are very alert during sleep, blinking frequently. In sleeping herring gulls, for example, the eyes are never closed for more than 60 seconds. However, at the physiological level, sleep in birds appears to be very different from mammalian sleep. There is no evidence, for example, that birds have REM sleep.

Summary of Section 2.5

1   The function of sleep is studied by looking at individual variation, by experimental manipulation of sleep, and by comparing sleep in different species. So far, such studies have confirmed that REM sleep may be important for brain development and sleep deprivation results in poor mental and physical performance.

2   The ancestral function of sleep may be to conserve energy and to keep animals out of harm's way at times of day when they might otherwise be at risk or unable to function effectively.

3   For humans, sleep allows the brain to recuperate and there is some evidence that it enhances memory formation and learning.

4   There is much variation in sleep patterns across species; the timing and duration of sleep in a particular species is adapted to that species' pattern of activity.

2.6 Sleep medicine

Many people suffer from a lack of sleep, or from very disturbed sleep. There are a number of irritating sleep 'disturbances'. The three most common are: sleep talking, snoring and bruxism (tooth grinding). The latter is particularly common in young children. A survey of more than 400 adults (aged 20–64) in Sweden revealed that 12% suffered from **persistent insufficient sleep (PIS)**; half of the people with PIS had additional sleep problems. The most common causes of PIS were work-related factors that allowed insufficient time for sleep (Broman et al., 1996). Many people with sleep problems seek their own remedy, such as drinking alcohol or buying sleeping pills from a pharmacy. Herbal remedies are particularly popular in some parts of the world and are used for sleep problems by 1 in 8 people in the USA. Sleeping problems are especially prevalent among the elderly; a Canadian study found that one in four elderly people used some kind of non-prescription drug, alcohol or herbal remedy to improve their sleep (Martin, 2002).

Many people with persistent sleep problems go to their doctor. Up until the 1970s, the typical treatment was the prescription of *barbiturate* drugs, the effect of which is to suppress the activity of the central nervous system. These were very unsatisfactory because they are long-lasting and impair daytime alertness and performance. They also create problems of their own, being physiologically and psychologically addictive and also dangerous; patients develop tolerance to barbiturates and require ever-larger doses to get to sleep; an overdose can be fatal. Addiction to barbiturates is called barbiturism; symptoms include confusion, slurred speech, yawning, sleepiness, memory loss, loss of balance and reduction in muscular reflexes. Drug withdrawal must be done slowly, over one to three weeks, to avoid withdrawal symptoms, such as tremors and convulsions, which can be fatal.

Barbiturates were replaced by *benzodiazepines*, such as Valium and Librium, which were developed to treat anxiety disorders. A problem with these is that, like alcohol, they stimulate the early REM stages of sleep at the expense of deep, slow-wave sleep. Modern hypnotic drugs are being developed that do not cause such problems.

● What would be the characteristics of the ideal sleeping drug?

● It would act quickly, so that it could be taken in immediate response to insomnia and does not have to be taken continuously; it should be short-acting, so that the patient does not feel drowsy during the day.

All drugs cause side-effects, and much sleep medicine research is aimed at finding non-pharmaceutical remedies to sleep disorders. **Cognitive behavioural therapy** (a form of therapy in which patients are helped to correct false perceptions about their relationship to the world) has proved very effective for some patients. Another ingenious technique, developed in Russia, involves the creation of individually designed 'brain music'. An insomniac's EEG brain patterns are recorded during sleep and are used as the basis of musical sounds that the patient can play to themselves when they want to sleep; this is effective for some people.

The key to finding an effective remedy for a sleep disorder is correct diagnosis. Sleep, as we have seen, is a complex phenomenon that is intimately linked to other physiological processes. A recent listing of sleep disorders identifies no less that 54 distinct conditions (Table 2.2); as research continues, this number is likely to increase.

A key feature of this classification is that it separates disorders that are due to mechanisms controlling sleep itself (intrinsic sleep disorders) from those that are associated with other systems in the body or to external factors. Clearly, if a sleep disorder is not due to a failure of sleep mechanisms but to something else, the remedy is to address the 'something else', not to prescribe sleeping pills. This is particularly true of those disorders (extrinsic and clock-related) that result from life-styles that are harmful to sleep, such as excessive alcohol intake and shift work. We will now look briefly at some of the disorders listed in Table 2.2.

Sleep apnoea

The commonest sleep disorder, apnoea, involves a pause in breathing of more than 10 seconds, which usually causes a person to wake up. Apnoea can be caused, either by a physical obstruction or by a failure of the brain mechanisms that maintain regular breathing during sleep (Book 3, Section 3.4.4). Sleep apnoea can only be diagnosed by overnight monitoring and is treated in a variety of ways, ranging from radical surgery, through lifestyle changes such as losing weight and drinking less alcohol, to the simple remedy of not sleeping on your back (see Case Report 2.1). Central sleep apnoea is a less common form of the disorder and (like sudden infant death syndrome) is classed as a parasomnia because breathing stops as a consequence of a failure of the brainstem to produce a coordinated rhythmic motor output.

Table 2.2   A classification of sleep disorders.

Categories	Sub-categories	Number of recognized disorders, with examples
dyssomnias (cause difficulty in getting to sleep or staying asleep, or excessive daytime sleepiness)	intrinsic sleep disorders	12 – narcolepsy, sleep apnoea, restless legs syndrome
	extrinsic sleep disorders	13 – disorders caused by food allergies, stimulants, alcohol, toxins
	circadian rhythm sleep disorders	6 – jet-lag, shiftwork sleep disorder, delayed and advanced sleep phase disorders
parasomnias (undesirable intrusions of behaviour or nervous system function during sleep)	arousal disorders	3 – sleepwalking
	sleep-wake transition disorders	4 – sleep talking
	parasomnias associated with REM sleep	6 – nightmares
	other parasomnias	10 – snoring, central sleep apnoea, sudden infant death syndrome
medical/psychiatric sleep disorders		disorders caused by a neurological deficit or by generalized anxiety disorder

Case Report 2.1 Sleep apnoea

Anil, a 50-year-old man, had been sleeping badly for several years. His wife Nim had strongly urged him to make an appointment to see his GP after reading an article in a magazine about snoring. For several years Anil had snored very loudly in his sleep and Nim found her sleep severely disrupted and was now threatening to leave the marital bed. Whilst Anil was the person directly affected, Nim felt that she also suffered and that this was a problem that should not be dismissed casually and certainly not with a joke.

Nim recognized from the magazine article a description of snoring that matched Anil's snoring pattern and which resulted in disturbed sleep for them both. She read that during sleep the pharangeal airway narrows in everyone because there is a reduction in dilator muscle tone. During sleep the pharynx and soft palate vibrate and when this goes beyond a certain point, snoring occurs. When the pharangeal airway narrows further, then snoring gets louder and inspiration of breath also becomes laboured. If narrowing of the airway continues and the pharynx completely obstructs then breathing stops. This is termed sleep apnoea and Nim found that when Anil stopped breathing she became agitated, waiting anxiously to hear his next breath. Nim also read in the magazine that when breathing is restricted the increased inspiratory effort is sensed by the brain and transient arousal ensues. A few of these arousals throughout the night do not matter, but when they occur many times the result is seriously affected sleep. For Anil this resulted in excessive sleepiness in the daytime and he found that his ability to concentrate on his work as an accountant was adversely affected. He was also aware that at home and on the road he was impaired and in addition he often felt irritable.

Anil made an appointment and saw his GP who noted that Anil was overweight. Anil had a collar size of 17 and on visual examination had a small pharynx. When questioned, Anil explained that he nodded off to sleep very easily during the daytime and this was more than mere tiredness. He was also aware of waking up in the night feeling as though he was choking. The GP said Anil probably remembered only a tiny proportion of the actual number of times this happened and that one of the commonest causes of snoring and indeed sleep apnoea, is being overweight. The extra fat in the neck compresses the throat, particularly when muscles are relaxed during sleep. The GP suggested that Anil should consider a weight-reducing diet and advised against drinking alcohol after 6 pm as this relaxes the upper airway muscles even more. Anil did not smoke so this was not a contributory factor and neither did he have a receding lower jaw (sometimes treated with a dental intra-oral device). Anil's tonsils were not enlarged and neither did he have hypothyroidism, both of which could adversely affect his airway. Because Anil had nasal stuffiness a nasal spray of Flixonase twice a day and Rinatec at night to reduce inflammation was prescribed. In addition, and in order to reduce nocturnal nasal congestion, the GP suggested using pillows under the head end of the mattress and one thick or two thin pillows on top of the mattress to maximize pharangeal size. If symptoms persisted referral to a specialist centre could be considered. Then a diagnosis of sleep apnoea could be explored and treatment, which is normally instantly effective, using a small electric pump connected to a nasal mask to produce continuous positive airway pressure (CPAP), can be recommended. Other treatment options include surgery for ENT (ear, nose and throat) problems, but Anil felt happy to explore more conservative approaches in the first instance.

Narcolepsy

Narcolepsy is an extreme tendency to fall asleep or suffer overwhelming sleepiness during the day. Narcoleptics are usually easily awoken and become fully alert. In some people narcolepsy takes the form of a complete loss of muscle tone (cataplexy); they simple fall into a heap on the floor, but may still be awake. One form of narcolepsy affects one in 2000 people and it appears to be caused by a sudden intrusion of REM sleep into wakefulness (recall that REM sleep involves complete relaxation of the muscles). In mice, dogs and humans, narcolepsy is associated with abnormally low levels of a neuropeptide called hypocretin (secreted by the hypothalamus). In dogs and mice, a single allele has been identified that results in low hypocretin levels; in humans, genetic factors are believed to cause an autoimmune response which destroys hypocretin-secreting cells in the brain. Narcolepsy can be treated with the drug Ritalin, controversially used to treat attention deficit disorder (ADD) in children. Interestingly, ADD may be associated with sleep problems.

Delayed and advanced sleep phase disorders

As discussed earlier, there is much variation among people in terms, not only of how long they sleep, but also in when they naturally want to sleep. The distinction between 'larks' and 'owls' can be manifested, in extreme forms, as two related sleep disorders (Case Report 2.2). **Advanced sleep phase disorder (ASPD)** occurs when phases of the daily sleep/wake cycle are advanced with respect to clock time. The sleep phase occurs well ahead of conventional bedtime and the tendency is for individuals to wake up early. **Delayed sleep phase disorder (DSPD)** is a condition where the clock hour at which sleep normally occurs is moved back in time within the daily sleep/wake cycle. The result is a delayed occurrence of sleep and a delayed waking time.

Case Report 2.2 Living with an unusual sleep pattern

By 8 pm, I am sleepy, but generally do not go to bed until 9. I routinely wake at 3 or 4 am, and am instantly alert and cannot go back to sleep. I get up and do 3 hours work before breakfast, a habit that has many advantages for me. By lunchtime, I am feeling tired, incapable of coherent thought and able only to carry out routine tasks; if I am at home, I take a half-hour nap and wake feeling refreshed. If I have to go to work all day, I am tired and irascible in the afternoon; going to a seminar at lunchtime or in the afternoon inevitably induces sleep. I am typically poor company in the evening and find parties boring and stressful. I have advanced sleep phase disorder (ASPD) and the natural period of my biological clock is considerably less than 24 hours; I am a 'lark'.

My father also was a very early riser and frequently fell asleep during the day. My pattern of sleep and work seems to be getting more marked as I get older; this seems partly due to my responding to what seems 'natural' for me, partly because I have taken the opportunity to read a great deal about sleep and circadian rhythms and to develop a routine that works for me.

I work a lot with John, who exemplifies delayed sleep phase disorder (DSPD). He has great difficulty getting to sleep and generally does so about the time I am getting up; he is an 'owl'. He works most effectively in the evening. Fortunately, we work in an organization that does not insist that we conform to strict 9 to 5 working hours and we ensure that we communicate effectively by arranging our meetings at lunchtime.

Case Report 2.2 shows that ASPD and DSPD need not be a serious problem for people who can adjust their work schedules to suit their unusual sleep patterns. Many people, however, have to keep regular working hours and have health problems as a result. People with DSPD tend to develop an accumulated sleep debt, which they can offset by sleeping a great deal at the weekend. Both conditions can be treated by light therapy, which involves sitting in front of a very bright light for an hour or two every day. This has the effect of altering the timing of the biological clock. People with DSPD can alleviate the condition by having light therapy in the morning, those with ASPD in the evening.

2.6.1 Sleep and shift work

Case Report 2.3 describes how shift work is incompatible with normal sleep patterns and, as a result, constitutes a major health risk. For example, a 15-year study of shift workers found that individuals who had worked shifts for 11 years or longer were twice as likely as day workers to develop heart disease. In those who had worked shifts for more than 15 years, the risk of heart disease was three times greater. Women who work night shifts for many years are up to 60% more likely to develop breast cancer; it has been suggested that this results from abnormal patterns of secretion of melatonin (Davis et al., 2001).

● What effect would working at night in well-lit premises have on melatonin secretion?

● Melatonin levels would be decreased.

It has been found (in studies of birds) that melatonin 'switches on' gonadotropin-inhibitory hormone (GnIH) (Ubuka et al., 2005).

● Assuming that melatonin has the same effect in humans, how would this affect the pattern of oestrogen secretion in women who worked night shifts?

● If the level of secretion of melatonin decreases, then GnIH will not be secreted and the secretion of gonadotropin-releasing hormone (GnRH) will be unchecked, so levels of oestrogen would rise (see Figure 3.10 in Book 2).

High levels of oestrogen are a risk factor for breast cancer.

2.6.2 Sleep and accidents

As we saw in Section 2.4.1, during the day people frequently fall asleep very briefly. Micro-sleeps often go unnoticed, especially if they are very short, and there is evidence that they are more likely to occur in people who are sleep-deprived, and in the afternoon, when people are typically less alert. Having a micro-sleep while driving a car at speed can have disastrous consequences. It is estimated that at least 10% of road accidents in the UK are caused by drivers falling asleep. On motorways and major trunk roads, this proportion rises to 15%. Sleep, like alcohol, is a major cause of road accidents.

Most road accidents occur at night, between 02:00 and 06:00, and in the afternoon, between 14:00 and 16:00. Fifty per cent of sleep-related road accidents involve young men, aged 18 to 30. To a certain extent, these figures reflect what we know about sleep, for example that micro-sleeps are more likely to occur in the afternoon.

Case Report 2.3   The experience of a night shift worker

Night duty is worked as part of internal rotation in the Accident and Emergency (A&E) Department where I work. This means I work approximately 7 nights every 6 weeks. (In the six weeks between my last two holidays, of 225 hours worked, a hundred were at night.) I expect to work 7 nights over two weeks – 4 nights one week and 3 the next. Mostly this is respected but I have to fight for this work configuration and recently worked 3 nights, followed by 2 weeks annual leave, 4 more nights, 2 weeks day duty, then 3 more nights.

Before I start night duty I stock up on food as if preparing for a siege. I buy food for the duration and carefully plan my main meals. I also try to clean the house as I know I will do no housework during the night duty spell. In fact the house becomes more and more untidy as the nights progress. I always make my bed up clean, as the thought of a freshly laundered bed after the first night cheers and sustains me.

On the day of the first shift I try to sleep in the afternoon and lie down between 1.30 and 2 pm, usually on the settee, sometimes on the bed. The radio remains on and I usually manage to doze. I get up about 4.30 pm, drink tea, and from 5–8 pm, prepare and eat my main meal, prepare my food for work and take a bath. Only on night duty do I bath rather than shower. There is no food in the hospital at night except for an unsatisfactory vending machine, so I take filled rolls, fruit and cake to work.

On my first night I leave for work at 8 pm; the shift starts at 8.45, and I arrive early. My departure gets gradually later as the week progresses. The shifts span 11 hours, for which we are paid 10 hours. We have two half-hour breaks which are taken in the department. Because the A&E Department has full lighting all night, staying awake is not too difficult.

However, between 5 and 7 am it becomes increasingly difficult and if I sit down, I find my eyes closing momentarily. If possible, I take my second break at this time and catnap for about ten minutes.

The effects that night duty have on me can be divided into social, physical and mental. Socially, I am unable to have any social life and become increasingly lonely, as all I do is sleep and work. When I get up in the evening I feel unable to do anything that is not essential for fear of becoming tired. Even making a phone call has to be limited to friends who understand about being cut short because of the time. Physically, I become prone to headaches, constipation, thirst, flatulence, bad breath, obsession with eating and disorders of balance. Mentally, I become irritable, lose empathy with patients, find it difficult to make decisions, suffer from thought block, and have feelings of dissociation.

When the shift is over I drive home. This is a dangerous procedure and, I believe, breaks the law. In order not to fall asleep, I often sit in the coffee room and doze for 10–15 minutes before leaving. Sometimes I pull in on the journey home and have a catnap. I drive with the window open, singing or talking out loud to myself in order to stay awake. When I get home I either go straight to bed or have a mug of camomile tea and toast. Then to bed at 9.30 am.

When I wake my first thought is how many hours have I slept. When I get up during the day to go to the toilet, which I always do, my thought is always, will I be able to get back to sleep again? When the night duty span is finished it takes at least two and usually five days to recover completely. For people who have never worked night duty, the best way to describe it is to compare night duty with jet-lag or being drunk. Only when we work nights do my colleagues and I become obsessed with how many hours sleep we have had.

● What other factor may be involved in the these patterns of occurrence of sleep-related road accidents?

● Speed. Driving speeds are higher at times of day when there is less traffic. Young men may drive faster than other drivers.

The incidence of road accidents also shows a seasonal effect, related in part to changing the clocks in spring and autumn. There is a statistically significant increase in accidents in the spring, when clocks are put forward; even the loss of one hour of sleep causes sleep deprivation and disturbance of sleep patterns. Paradoxically, there is a similar effect when clocks are put back, allowing people an extra hour of sleep. Analysis of 21 years of data in the USA showed a significant increase in road fatalities at the end of daylight-saving time. It is thought that the explanation for this is that, anticipating an extra hour in bed, people tend to stay up later and to drink more alcohol.

Summary of Section 2.6

1   Insomnia, sleep deprivation and other sleep disorders are common in the human population and represent a major challenge to health services.

2   While many people use a wide variety of medications and herbal remedies to offset sleep problems, many sleep disorders can be solved by people adjusting their lives appropriately.

3   Certain aspects of modern life, such as shift-work and air travel, are a significant cause of sleep disorders.

2.7 Coda: towards a more rational lifestyle

'Tired people are stupid and reckless'

(Martin, 2002)

Insufficient sleep and poor quality sleep are a major cause of unhappiness, poor-health and accidents in modern human societies. These problems could largely be avoided if everyone got the amount of sleep that they need. The importance of adequate sleep is recognized in the regulations governing the working conditions of certain groups of people, notably airline pilots and drivers of trucks, buses and trains. In much of society, however, it is ignored and many people have to conform to work regimes that reduce their effectiveness, impair their health and increase the risk of accidents to themselves and to others. This is particularly true of junior hospital doctors in the UK (see British Medical Association, 2004).

The diaries of Alan Clark, former cabinet minister, provide an extraordinary picture of the higher levels of government, in which ministers, their advisors and senior civil servants are chronically sleep-deprived. Former Prime Minister Margaret Thatcher, who reputedly slept for only two hours each night, used to terrorize her ministers by phoning them at all hours of the night. There is a perception that being able to get by on little sleep is somehow admirable. There is also a perception that we can train ourselves to sleep less, or to sleep as and when we chose. This seems not to be true. Attempts to train the crews of US nuclear missile submarines to conform to highly abnormal sleep/wake patterns (a disturbing thought given their occupation) were a complete failure. The 24-hour biological clock and the diurnal cycle of sleep appear to be highly resistant to change. As our understanding of sleep and biological clocks increases, society should take heed and organize itself so that we all get sufficient sleep.

Questions for Chapter 2

Question 2.1 (LO 2.1)

Why is REM sleep also called paradoxical sleep?

Question 2.2 (LO 2.2)

What are the characteristics of deep sleep, and when does it occur?

Question 2.3 (LO 2.3)

You have spent some time in America and have just come home to find yourself falling asleep at odd times of day and waking up during the night. Why is this? How long will this situation last?

Question 2.4 (LO 2.4)

What changes occur in our sleep patterns as we get older?

Question 2.5 (LO 2.5)

Distinguish between the restorative and ecological theories for the function of sleep.

Question 2.6 (LO 2.6)

What is advanced sleep phase disorder (ASPD)?

Question 2.7 (LO 2.7)

Among animals, predators, such as cats and dogs, sleep a lot; herbivores, such as cows and horses, sleep much less. What does this suggest about the function of sleep?

References and Further Reading

References

Baehr, E. K., Revelle, W. and Eastman, C. I. (2000) Individual differences in the phase and amplitude of the human circadian temperature rhythm: with an emphasis on morningness-eveningness. *Journal of Sleep Research*, **9**, 117–127.

Bastien, C. H. and Morin, C. M. (2000) Familial incidence of insomnia. *Journal of Sleep Research*, **9**, 49–54.

Brain Briefings (1998) Adenosine and Sleep, Society for Neuroscience, May 1998.

British Medical Association (2004) [online]: Available from: http://www.bma.org.uk/ap.nsf/Content/HospitalDoctorsJunHrs (Accessed March 2005)

Broman, J. E., Lundh, L. G. and Hetta, J. (1996) Insufficient sleep in the general population. *Neurophysiologie Clinique*, **26**, 30–39.

Compact Oxford English Dictionary (1996) Oxford: Oxford University Press.

Davis, S., Mirick, D. K. and Stevens, R. G., (2001) Night shift work, light at night, and risk of breast cancer. *Journal of the National Cancer Institute*, **93**, 1557–1562.

Gaudreau, H., Carrier, J. and Montplaisir, J. (2001) *Journal of Sleep Research*, **10**, 165–172.

Guyton, A. C. and Hall, J. E. (1996) *Textbook of Medical Physiology*, 9th edn. Philadelphia: W. B. Saunders.

Krueger, J. M., Obal, J. F. and Fang, J. (1999) Humoral regulation of physiological sleep: cytokines and GHRH. *Journal of Sleep Research*, **8**, 53–59.

Martin, P. (2002) *Counting Sheep*. London: Harper Collins.

Mednick, S. C., Nakayama, K. and Stickgold, R. (2003) Sleep-dependent learning: a nap is as good as a night. *Nature Neuroscience*, **6**, 697–698.

Siegel, J. M. (2001) The REM sleep-memory consolidation hypothesis. *Science*, **294**, 1058–1063.

Spiegel, K., Leproult, R. and Van Cauter, E. (1999) Impact of sleep debt on metabolic and endocrine function. *Lancet*, **354**, 1435–1439.

Stores, G. and Wiggs, L. (2001) *Sleep Disturbance in Children and Adolescents with Disorders of Development – its Significance and Management*. Cambridge: Cambridge University Press.

Taillard, J., Philip, P., Coste, O., Sagaspe, P. and Bioulac, B. (2003) The circadian and homeostatic modulation of sleep pressure during wakefulness differs between morning and evening chronotypes. *Journal of Sleep Research*, **12**, 275–282.

Ubuka, T., Bentley, G. E., Ukena, K., Wingfield, J. C. and Tsutsui, K. (2005) Melatonin induces the expression of gonadotropin-inhibitory hormone in the avian brain. *Proceedings of the National Academy of Sciences, USA*, **102**, 3052–3057.

Vitkovic, L., Bockaert, J. and Jacque, C. (2000) 'Inflammatory' cytokines: neuromodulators in normal brain? *Journal of Neurochemistry*, **74**, 457–471.

Wirtz-Justice, A. (1998) Beginning to see the light. *Archives of General Psychiatry*, **55**, 860–862.

Wirz-Justice, A., Krauchi, K. and Wirz, H. (1991) Season, gender and age: interaction with sleep and nap timing and duration in an epidemiological survey in Switzerland. Abstract, World Federation of Sleep Research Societies Congress.

Yoon, I-Y., Kripke, D. F., Youngstedt, S. D. and Elliott, J. A. (2003) Actigraphy suggests age-related differences in napping and nocturnal sleep. *Journal of Sleep Research*, **12**, 87–93.

Zhdanova, I. V., Wurtman, R. J., Morabito, C., Piotrivska, V. R. and Lynch, H. J. (1996) Effect of low oral doses of melatonin, given 2–4 hours before habitual bedtime, on sleep in normal young humans. *Sleep*, **19**, 423–432.

Further Reading

Science (2001), **294**, pp. 1048–1063.

STRESS

3.1 Introduction

Working for the British Civil Service is not most people's idea of a stressful life. Civil servants are the officials and administrators who run the government's various departments and agencies. The Civil Service is acknowledged to be a good employer, providing pension benefits, relatively secure employment, pleasant London offices, and so on. Britain's National Health Service is freely available for all civil service employees. Though there is variation in income within the service, no-one is on poverty pay (and no-one is becoming a millionaire).

Let us carry out a thought experiment, then. The Civil Service is divided up into numerous grades of employee, from secretaries and clerical support staff through to heads of department and executives. Let us imagine that we took a large sample of middle-aged employees who were all healthy, and followed them for around eight years, to see which ones developed heart disease. Some of the participants were low-grade staff, some intermediate, and some were in high-grade positions. At the end of the study period, which of them would be most likely to have had heart problems?

There are several possible hypotheses. The most obvious one is that there would be no relationship between people's grade of employment and their risk of heart disease. This seems to make sense. All participants worked for the same employer in the same city. All participants were well above the poverty line. All did work in an office environment. All had access to health care. Whatever it was that made some people vulnerable to heart disease – genetics, diet, exercise – would not be systematically related to their grade within the service, so overall, no pattern would be detectable.

An alternative hypothesis would be that the higher the grade of the service held, the greater the risk of heart disease. People at the top have heavy responsibilities for decisions that affect millions of people. They must suffer overwork and 'executive stress' – enough to give anyone a heart attack. Thus, under this hypothesis, you would expect to find a higher proportion of heart disease cases in the higher grades.

Finally, there is the alternative possibility. People in the lower grades have to take orders from everyone else. They turn up and put in their hours like everyone else, but the rewards are lower and the power they hold is less. Perhaps they will be the ones at highest risk.

The study we have described here has been carried out. In fact, two such studies have been performed. The one described here is the second. Michael Marmot and his colleagues at University College London contacted over ten thousand civil servants in the late 1980s, and screened them for existing heart disease, as well as finding out about their jobs and life-styles. Over the next eight years or so, they monitored them to see who developed heart problems. The problems they recorded were: heart attack (a fairly unmistakable outcome), angina (the crushing pressure in the chest felt when the heart is not getting enough oxygen), and other severe chest pains.

● How would you describe these events?

◉ These would be termed coronary heart disease (CHD) events (Book 3, Section 2.6.2).

Returning to the three possible hypotheses above (no relationship, more CHD in the higher grades, more CHD in the lower grades), think about which one is likely to have been correct, and why that might be. The results of the study, and possible explanations, are considered below.

Some of the data from the study are reproduced in Table 3.1. The greatest number of cases of CHD is in the intermediate grades of employment.

● Does this mean that the risk of CHD is highest in the intermediate grades?

◉ Not necessarily, because the number of participants from the intermediate grade is larger than the other two. You would expect the raw number of cases to be higher even if the risk was the same.

Table 3.1 Numbers of cases of CHD (coronary heart disease) in the Whitehall II study, by employment grade.

Grade	Number of participants	Number of cases of CHD
Higher	2037	163
Intermediate	3086	290
Lower	1074	142

To calculate the risk, the first step is to consider not the absolute number of cases, but the proportion of people in each category who have developed CHD.

● From Table 3.1, what is the proportion of people in each category developing CHD?

● Higher grades: 163 / 2037 = 0.080 or 8%

   Intermediate: 290 / 3086 = 0.094 or 9.4%

   Lower grades   142 / 1074 = 0.132 or 13.2%

The data thus show that the civil servants in the highest grades have the lowest risk of CHD, and those in the lowest grade have the highest risk. Of course, further controls need to be made. People in the lower grades are younger and tend to be women, whereas those in the higher grades are older and tend to be men. Age and sex will independently affect risk of heart disease. When the researchers controlled for these other factors, the results were even more striking; the higher your grade in the civil service, the lower your risk of having a heart attack.

● Can you think of any factors (other than stress, which we discuss in detail in the rest of the chapter) which might explain the pattern observed?

● It could be the case that lower grade employees have poorer diets, smoke and drink more, take less physical exercise, or are more obese.

The researchers were naturally concerned to locate the causes of the pattern that they have found, and so they measured and controlled for life-style factors that they could identify. The lower grade employees did indeed smoke more, and were a little less physically active. However, the differences were not sufficient to explain the increased risk of CHD. Their blood cholesterol (which is correlated with the risk of developing atherosclerosis) and their body mass index (BMI), a measure of body composition which can be an index of obesity (Book 1, Section 3.2.2), were roughly the same as measurements in the highest grades. Thus there is an unexplained factor that differs between different grades within the same organization and that makes some employees more likely than others to have a heart attack. This factor is very likely to be related to stress, and in this chapter, we will be finding out what stress is, and why it has the effects that it does.

3.2 The concept of stress

It is very tempting to explain the increase in coronary heart disease in the low grades of the civil service by calling in the concept of *stress*. We could say that because the low-graders were subject to more stress, their health deteriorated. The problem with this explanation is that we have not specified what stress is. If by stress we mean just 'prone to bad health', then all we have said is that the low-graders were prone to more bad health because they were prone to more bad health. The concept will only be meaningful if we can identify a specific chain of causality running from the conditions of being a low-grade employee to the outcome of heart disease.

This is not easy to do. The differences between the Civil Service grades are not noticeable in the objective physical conditions of their work. It is not as if high grades work in pleasant office buildings in a green neighbourhood whilst low grades work in noisy and dangerous mines surrounded by pollution. All grades work the

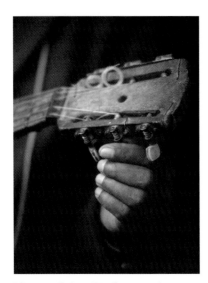

Figure 3.1 Tuning a guitar string by exerting stress upon it.

same hours in the same buildings in the same city. It is their *psychological* experience – of being a boss versus being a cog in the machine – which is so different. Heart disease, on the other hand, is caused by the formation of plaques that reduce the efficiency of the delivery of blood to tissues (including the tissue of the heart itself), and can lead to the heart stopping. Plaque formation is clearly a *physiological* event, although the underlying cause is not known (Book 3, Section 2.6.2). So the question is: what process could possibly link *psychological* experience with *physiological* outcomes? What intermediate steps does such a linkage go through, and why does it happen? This is an even more interesting question, since the lower grade employees don't just have more heart disease. They have more illness of many kinds, and a shorter life expectancy. The different maladies for which they and groups like them have an elevated risk of suffering involve the immune system, the nervous system, the digestive system, and the reproductive system, as well as the cardiovascular system. What process, originating largely in the mind, could possibly have such widespread effects?

The concept of stress comes from engineering. Consider a guitar string, held taut by its tuning peg (Figure 3.1). When the string is loose, tightening the peg by one turn just causes the string to stretch a little. But when the string is already very tight, turning the peg one turn more can make the string suddenly snap. The increase in tension is the same in both cases, but in the latter condition the string was already under *stress*, which meant that a little change was enough to cause a failure, a failure with severe consequences.

It is easy to see the metaphorical parallel between that string and how we feel when we have a lot of things going against us, but the physiological usage of the word stress is actually very specific. The pioneers of the use of the concept of stress in biology were Walter Cannon (1871–1945) and Hans Selye (1907–1982). Their development of the concept derives from experiments conducted on animals, mainly rats. To this day, much of the work on the physiology of stress is carried out on laboratory animals. Naturally, there are both ethical and scientific issues surrounding such work. By definition, stress is unpleasant and involves subjecting the animals to conditions they would naturally avoid. On the other hand, the investigations carried out on animals are of a type that could not be done with human volunteers, but sometimes lead to applications which do benefit humans. One branch of stress research has also benefited animals, too, since research on stress helps to design optimal conditions for keeping livestock and captive animals.

In his original experiments, Selye noticed that rats which were subjected to certain laboratory procedures underwent a suite of physiological changes. The adrenal gland was enlarged, and tissues of the immune system (such as the thymus, where many immune cells are produced) were shrunken.

● Where is the adrenal gland situated, and what are its functions?

● The adrenal gland is situated on top of the kidney. It secretes several important hormones into the bloodstream, e.g. corticosteroids, such as cortisol and mineralocorticoids, such as aldosterone (Book 2, Box 3.1) from the adrenal cortex. Adrenalin is secreted from the adrenal medulla.

● In the context of a physiological response to stress, which cells of the thymus would you expect to proliferate?

● The white cells, known as T cells (Book 2, Section 3.8; Book 3, Section 4.5.4).

The rats often developed stomach ulcers. This is significant because ulcers are often found also in people who have been through periods of emotional strain. Selye felt that it was not the content of the experiments being done on the rats that was causing these changes, but, rather, the very experience of being experimented on. To show this, he needed to run a control group.

● What is a control group, and of what would such a group consist in this case?

● In experimental science, a control group is a group that receives exactly the same treatment as the experimental group in every respect *except* for the variable whose effect is being studied (Book 1, Section 2.12). In this case, a good control group would be a group of rats kept in the same cages under the same conditions, but not taken out to participate in experiments.

The control group stayed in their cages all day and showed none of the features that the experimental group had shown. Subsequent experiments revealed the types of factor that induced the syndrome that Selye had discovered in the rat. The same changes result from holding them immobile, constantly changing their environments, overcrowding them or exposing them to a predator. Moreover, the effects are broader than those initially noted by Selye. Prolonged stress reduces life expectancy, increases cardiovascular problems, slows the rate of growth, can upset reproductive cycles, affects learning and memory, and even increases susceptibility to infectious disease. Selye called what he had observed the *general adaptation syndrome*, which meant that there were a suite of different changes in the environment that could cause the syndrome, and a suite of physiological responses that ensued. We would now call the general adaptation syndrome the **stress response**. Over the years we have come to understand the physiology of the stress response, in both humans and other animals, fairly well, as we shall find out in the next section.

Whatever the ethical issues, animal experiments have been fruitful in stress research, for two reasons. The first is that the stress response has the peculiar property that, though the causes of stress are extremely varied (malnutrition, receiving injections, being shouted at), they all tend to activate pretty much the same physiological mechanisms. The consequences (peptic ulcers, heart attacks, and so on) are also very varied. However, once again, there is a small number of physiological mechanisms that feed into all these different effects. The stress response is thus a kind of common pathway between a whole load of different environmental factors, and a whole set of different outcomes in the body (Figure 3.2 overleaf). This means that doing experiments on the effects of, for example, 'overcrowding stress' in the rat, can be generalized to the effects of say, 'stress through noise'.

The second convenient feature of the stress response is that its biology is highly conserved. This means that the physiological mechanisms are very similar in related species, and thus probably can be traced back, relatively unchanged, to a common ancestor species. It turns out that the stress response works in very

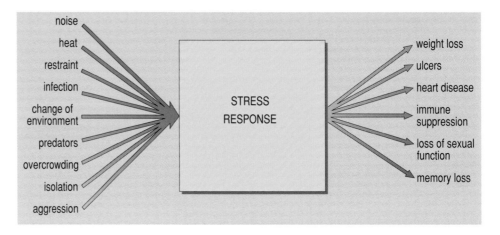

Figure 3.2   The stress response as a common pathway between multiple causes and multiple effects in the rat.

similar ways in mice, rats, tree shrews, monkeys and humans. Of course, the kinds of things that are stressors differ from species to species, as well as differing between individuals, but the physiological effects of stress are largely the same. This means that when scientists do experiments on one species, they can make inferences about how the system will work in other species as well, thus speeding up the rate of progress in understanding. Much of the research we will review has been carried out on rats, mice and monkeys. There are obviously issues of both science and ethics surrounding the use of such animals, and you may wish to consider what these are as you continue with the chapter.

Summary of Section 3.2

1   The concept of stress was originally introduced to explain changes in the body – such as shrunken immune tissue and ulcer formation – that resulted from changes in the experience of experimental animals.

2   The stress response system is similar in humans and non-human mammals.

3   The stress response is a common pathway which links many different kinds of environmental or psychological events with many different physiological outcomes.

3.3 Physiology of the stress response

In this section, we will be discovering what the immediate effect of a stressful situation (known as a **stressor**) is on the body. Because of the features of the stress response described above (its generality and its conservation), we could look at the response of humans or rats, and choose from a variety of stressors and our observations would be valid. In humans, the stress response has been shown to be provoked by stimuli as diverse as exams, public speaking, combat, mental arithmetic tests, medical procedures, and thinking about difficult problems (Figure 3.3).

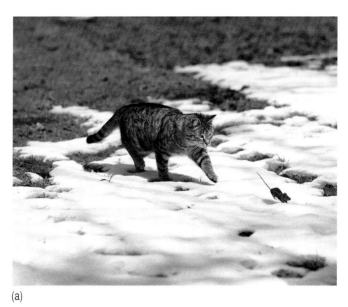

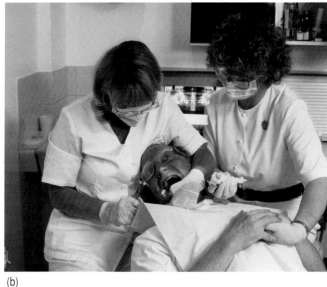

(a)   (b)

Figure 3.3   Stressors will be somewhat different for (a) mice and (b) humans.

The following example of an investigation of stress is from a recent study of women undergoing gynaecological surgery (Migneault et al., 2004). The researchers were investigating whether playing relaxing music during surgery would reduce the physiological signs of stress. (It did not.) However, here we are not concerned with the actual hypothesis of the study, but with the workings of the stress response, so we will concentrate on what happened to their control group (the ones not hearing any music, but who were going through the surgery nonetheless). The study has a number of useful features. First, the women were definitely under extreme stress, so the physiological response is very clear.

● How would you describe this stress?

● They were all undergoing the same medical procedure, so you could say that the physical stressor was the same in each case. You might also have reflected that the women's emotional states prior to anaesthesia may have differed wildly but the point at which measurements began was post-anaesthesia.

Second, because the women were immobilized on a surgical table for the whole of the experience, and already having their physiology closely monitored, it was easy for the researchers to gather data on exactly how their bodies were responding.

Measurements were taken at four points during the surgery. At phase 1, the women were lying in theatre and had just received oxygen and an anaesthetic through a mask. They were gradually passing out. Note that being unconscious does not eliminate the stress response. The surgery then began, and phase 2 was defined as 5 minutes after the first incision. Phase 3 was the point at which the incision finished being stitched. Finally, phase 4 was 30 minutes later than phase 3, when the women were recovering in an area outside the operating theatre.

We shall now look at the different physiological components of the stress response and see how and why these are triggered.

3.3.1 The circulatory system

First, let us examine the changes occurring in the blood circulatory system of these women (Figure 3.4). Note that the blood pressure rises with the first surgical incision and continues to rise throughout the procedure. The heart rate increases (tachycardia) at the beginning of the operation, but stabilizes and gradually returns to baseline with time. Note that the small size of the increase during the operation is partly a by-product of the anaesthetic in this case; if someone was doing something very stressful to you without anaesthesia, the chances are that your heart rate would go considerably higher than 78 beats per minute!

Figure 3.4 Women's blood pressure and heart rate throughout an abdominal surgical procedure.

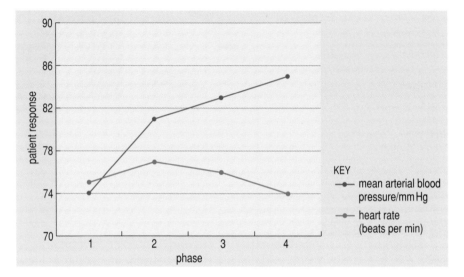

Why do heart rate and blood pressure increase? On detection of a stressor (tissue damage), the brain sends out signals through the autonomic nervous system (ANS) to effect certain physiological changes. At this point, you might want to briefly recap on the nervous system from Book 2, Chapter 1. You will recall that the peripheral nervous system (the part that extends beyond the brain and spinal cord into the rest of the body) can be divided into somatic and autonomic pathways.

● What are the functions of the somatic and autonomic nervous systems?

● The somatic system controls voluntary movements, such as picking up a cup. The autonomic nervous system is a separate set of connections that regulates all those involuntary activities of which you are scarcely aware, such as breathing and heart beat, but which require continual small adjustments according to the situation.

The autonomic nervous system is further divided into two branches, whose connections work antagonistically (see Figure 1.16 in Book 2).

● What are the two branches of the autonomic nervous system called?

● The sympathetic and parasympathetic nervous systems.

● Which branch of the ANS is responsible for increasing the heart rate, and which neurotransmitter does it use?

● When the sympathetic nervous system releases noradrenalin the heart beats faster.

●   From which region of the brain do sympathetic signals to the heart originate?

●   From the vasomotor centre in the medulla (Book 3, Section 2.4.6; see also Figure 2.7 there).

The sympathetic nervous system also innervates the circular, smooth muscle rings surrounding the arteries, causing them to contract, forcing the arteries to narrow and blood to circulate at a higher rate (because, of course, a given amount of liquid pumping round smaller tubes is going to go faster). Muscles around the lungs relax, meaning that the capacity of the lungs is increased. Whilst the circulation is gearing up to work harder, other systems are slowed down. Signals from the sympathetic nervous system cause the muscular contractions that are always going on in the stomach and intestines to decrease. This is the classic 'fright, fight or flight' response (Book 2, Section 1.8.2; Book 3, Section 2.4.6). The parasympathetic nervous system has the complementary functions to the sympathetic. When signals come down these pathways, the heartbeat is slowed, the arteries dilate, and the stomach and intestines resume their work of digestion.

Following perception of a stressor, the brain sends of a volley of nerve impulses out through the sympathetic nervous system, increasing heart rate and blood pressure, and stopping digestive work. Because of the complementary functioning of sympathetic and parasympathetic pathways, parasympathetic activity goes down in response to a stressor just as sympathetic activity goes up.

3.3.2 Hormonal changes

Signalling from brain to body in response to stress is carried out not just by direct neural connections, but also by hormones. Recall the difference between neural and hormonal signalling. Neural signals involve an electrical potential (action potential) travelling down a neural fibre to a particular location. For example, the brain can send a signal to the heart muscle through a specific bundle of neurons that runs to the chest. Neural signalling is fast and reaches a specific target efficiently – like sending an email to someone whose address you know.

By contrast, hormonal signalling involves the brain contacting glands that release certain hormones into the blood. No cell in the body is further than four cells away from a blood vessel, and so hormones can reach a very wide variety of tissues. It is a slower business than sending a specific neural signal, since hormones take some time to circulate and diffuse, but it has the advantage of being a broadcast system. In a state of national emergency, information would be sent out over the radio, rather than emailed to specific individual citizens, and so where there are actions required from many different groups of cells, hormonal signalling is more effective.

Activity in the sympathetic nervous system causes the adrenal glands (situated on top of the kidneys; see Book 2, Figure 3.5) to release a hormone, adrenalin. Other tissues adjacent to sympathetic nerve endings in distributed sites throughout the body release a closely related hormone called noradrenalin.

Adrenalin and noradrenalin are at least partly responsible for the metabolic changes in the various organs described so far – for this reason, we often describe a sudden change in heart rate and arousal as 'an adrenalin rush'. Adrenalin is also responsible for the rapid mobilization of glucose reserves to provide energy for these emergency 'fright, fight or flight' situations. Returning to the women's surgery study, the researchers monitored blood levels of adrenalin and noradrenalin in the patients, and we can see that these have started to increase by phase 2, and increase steadily throughout the surgical procedure (Figure 3.5).

As well as the release of adrenalin and noradrenalin, the perception of a stressor causes another hormonal cascade event, which you have already encountered briefly in Book 2, Section 3.5.2. The brain region called the hypothalamus signals to the nearby anterior pituitary, which in turn releases a hormone called ACTH (adrenocorticotropic hormone) into the circulation. The main function of ACTH is to signal to the adrenal glands to begin releasing cortisol into the circulation. This system is called the HPA (hypothalamic-pituitary-adrenal) axis. It is in many ways a curious system. A stressor causes a fast, direct signal from the brain to the adrenal medulla to stimulate adrenalin release, and also a slower, indirect HPA signal to the same organ, but different region (cortex), to stimulate cortisol release. The different pathways probably reflect the fact that adrenalin and cortisol have rather different functions in the stress response, as we shall see.

Figure 3.5 Blood levels of adrenalin, noradrenalin, ACTH and cortisol during an abdominal surgical procedure. Adrenalin, noradrenalin and cortisol are on the left axis, ACTH on the right axis.

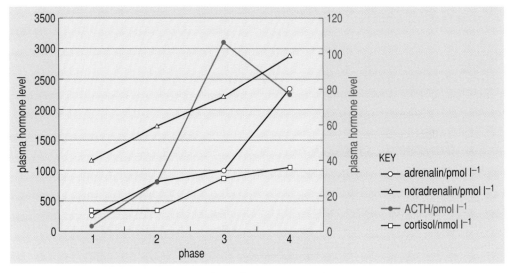

As you can see from Figure 3.5, in the women undergoing surgery, both ACTH and cortisol blood levels increased. The time course of the hormone release was subtly different for the different hormones, and it is worth looking at this closely.

● Describe and interpret the time-course of changing hormone levels for adrenalin and noradrenalin, ACTH and cortisol.

◐ Adrenalin and noradrenalin levels have already increased significantly by phase 2 (5 minutes after first incision), and they continue to increase until the end of the observations. ACTH levels have started to increase by phase 2, but have their maximum rate of increase between phases 2 and 3. Cortisol levels have not increased at all by phase 2, but rise somewhat later than the other hormones, between phases 2 and 3, presumably in response to the increased blood levels of ACTH.

The slower response rate of cortisol release compared to the other hormones reflects its different role. Whereas the actions of adrenalin and the sympathetic nervous system are principally concerned with mounting an emergency response – preparing the heart to supply the blood to the muscles, and so on – cortisol, and a suite of related hormones associated with it, seem more concerned with fuelling continued heightened action, as we shall see in the next section.

3.3.3 Metabolism

The body requires energy to work, and tissues that are working obtain this energy by metabolizing glucose and fats. These are stored in the body in various ways.

● Where are the principal depots of these metabolites and in what form are they stored?

● Fats are stored in adipocytes within adipose tissue as triglycerols (Book 1, Section 3.4). Glucose is stored as glycogen in hepatocytes within liver tissue, and it is also stored in skeletal muscles (Book 1, Section 3.3).

● Which hormone facilitates the uptake of glucose and its conversion to glycogen?

● The formation of glycogen is stimulated by insulin. High blood levels of insulin promote the uptake of glucose from the blood into the target tissues, which convert it into glycogen (Book 2, Section 3.7.1).

● In which human disease is the insulin system not working properly, and what are the consequences of such a malfunction?

● Diabetes mellitus. For various reasons (either the body does not produce enough insulin, or tissues are unresponsive to the insulin it does produce), the insulin-mediated mechanism fails and glucose is not removed from the circulation. Blood glucose levels can become dangerously high, leading to an event known as a hyperglycaemic episode (Book 2, Section 3.7.2).

Cortisol, along with glucagon, a hormone that, like insulin, is secreted by the pancreas (glucagon from the α cells of the islets of Langerhans; insulin from the β cells) acts in a contrary manner to insulin (insulin levels themselves are also lowered during stress). That is to say, tissues respond to cortisol and glucagon by breaking down glycogen into glucose and releasing it into the blood stream. Fat cells break down triglycerols into fatty acids and release them into the blood. Thus the blood becomes more energy rich for any tissues that require energy to do work. The cortisol response seems designed to fuel an ongoing bout of vigorous activity such as running away (Book 2, Section 3.7.1).

3.3.4 Pain, reproduction, and the immune system

There are also other consequences of the stress response that were not monitored during the women's surgery study. First, levels of reproductive hormones such as oestrogen, progesterone and testosterone are generally reduced during stressful situations, reducing sexual and reproductive performance. The consequences of this will be discussed in the next section.

Second, a class of compounds called the **endorphins** is released from the pituitary gland. The endorphins are notorious because they act at the same neurotransmitter receptors as the drugs opium, heroin and morphine (or perhaps that should be the other way around, opium, heroin and morphine are notorious because of their relationship to the functioning of the body's own endorphins). One consequence of the endorphin release is that sensitivity to painful stimuli is reduced. As well as explaining why morphine is used to treat severe pain, this explains why people who have been injured in battle or accidents manage to overcome their pain and drag themselves to safety – the endorphin blunts the pain and helps them to function and survive.

The stress response also affects the immune system. The linkage is both controversial and complex, as we shall see, but it can be clearly demonstrated. For example, let us consider some experiments using a rat model (Wiegers et al., 1993). Rats in these experiments had their adrenal glands removed, so that they could not produce any stress hormones naturally. This meant that the researchers could control the blood levels of stress hormones in the animals without any interference from the animals' natural production.

Recall that the immune system attacks pathogens, such as bacteria and viruses, entering the body, using a wide array of circulating specialized cells or lymphocytes. In the study described here, the focus was particularly on T-cells, which mature in the thymus and are released into the bloodstream where they play a role in immobilizing and destroying pathogens (Book 3, Section 4.5.4).

The experiments involved injecting the animals with a protein called concavalin. In normal animals, concavalin has the effect of stimulating the rate of cell division of T-cells. In this respect, it can be seen as a kind of simulation of a pathogen, since pathogens also stimulate T-cell division in the thymus. The researchers found that the proliferation of T-cells in response to the concavalin challenge varied according to the presence of corticosterone (the rat equivalent of the hormone cortisol) (see Figure 3.6).

In Figure 3.6, condition 1 represents control animals with natural levels of corticosterone and condition 2 represents adrenalectomized rats. Since their adrenals have been removed, the rats in this latter group have almost no circulating stress hormones.

● How would you describe their T-cell proliferation compared to the control group (condition 1)?

◐ Their T-cell response is much diminished, to less than half that of the control group.

Condition 3 is a group of rats that are adrenalectomized, but have been given a 12.5 mg pellet of corticosterone intravenously.

● What is the effect of administering corticosterone to these adrenalectomized rats?

◐ The corticosterone treatment returns the immune cell response to about 9.5, i.e. almost to the level of just above 10, as seen in the control group).

Finally, condition 4 is a group of rats that have been given a much higher dose of corticosterone (a 100 mg pellet).

● What is the response to this very much higher dose of replacement corticosterone?

◐ The immune response is almost completely abolished, at about 1.5, a level below that of the rats with no corticosterone at all.

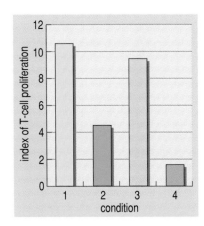

Figure 3.6 T-cell proliferation in response to a concavalin challenge. For the different conditions, see text.

● What does the pattern of results shown in Figure 3.6 suggest about the relationship between cortisol/corticosterone and immune activity?

● The results suggest that low concentrations of steroid hormone facilitate the immune response, but that very high concentrations begin to suppress it.

The interpretation of such results that has become popular in recent years is that the immediate effect of a stressor is to enhance immune system activity by causing an increase in activity and signalling amongst immune cells. It has been shown with experimental animals that exposure to an infection itself causes a stress response, which makes sense if the stress response is partly mobilizing the immune system's resources. Suppression of the immune system by the high dose of corticosterone will be discussed in Section 3.4.

3.3.5 The brain

Perhaps the most intriguing and controversial set of linkages is that between the stress response and the brain. Activity in the sympathetic nervous system makes us feel alert, aware and vigilant. We all recognize how a stressful occasion makes sensation particularly vivid and memorable. For example, people can often remember in unusual detail what they were doing at the time they heard the news of some terrible event. Intuitively, it seems that the stress response enhances the formation of memories. But is there any good evidence that this actually happens?

A number of studies have shown that consumption of glucose around the time of memorizing a stimulus, like a story or list of words, improves the memory for that stimulus (e.g. Gold, 1986). Further evidence comes from a study in which participants had to remember as much as they could from a story that they read (Cahill et al., 1994). The story came in two versions, which were very similar, but crucial paragraphs were altered so that the content was distressing in one case and neutral in the other. For example, in the neutral version, a boy passes a hospital where staff are practising for an emergency, and their various procedures are described. In the distressing version, the boy is critically injured in an accident, and the medical staff are doing the same things, but are now really fighting to save the boy, who has had his feet severed amongst other horrific injuries.

Unsurprisingly, the distressing version is remembered much more accurately than the neutral version, presumably because reading the stressful version elicits a stress response in the listener, which includes the release of extra blood glucose. The researchers then tried the same experiment where the participants had previously been given a drug called a beta-blocker.

● What do beta-blockers block?

● They block $\beta1$- and $\beta2$-adrenoceptors (Book 3, Section 2.6.1).

● For which chemical are adrenoceptors receptors?

● They are receptors for adrenalin and noradrenalin.

For groups of participants who had taken a beta-blocker, there was no difference in recall between the neutral and the distressing versions. Interestingly, though, the subjects still rated the distressing version as more distressing than the neutral one. Their subjective experience was affected by the gore just like those individuals who took no beta-blocker. However, the memory advantage of the distressing version was gone.

● How do you interpret the results of this study?

● The participants who read the distressing version perceived it as stressful, and probably initiated a stress response in both the beta-blocker and the no-drug conditions. In the no-drug condition, the stress response went through its normal cascade, effecting a range of physiological changes, including glucose release (see Section 3.3.2). In the beta-blocker condition, the stress response was blocked by the insensitivity of the body to rising adrenalin levels, and so although there was a psychological experience of distress, it could not initiate the full set of consequential effects that it normally would.

The mechanisms by which the stress response provides a memory advantage are not fully understood; glucose levels may be only one factor in a much more complex system of brain chemistry interactions. However, it seems likely that the adrenalin effect confers some advantage in stressful situations, probably by increasing alertness and danger recognition.

You may be aware that, as well as being a useful treatment for high blood pressure, beta-blockers are also used to treat panic and anxiety symptoms. [The stress response can sometimes be so extreme that it leads to a panic attack (see Case Report 3.1), but usually it is much less extreme.] Beta-blockers are effective because they block the effects of adrenalin, but the caveats mentioned in Section 2.6.1 of Book 3 can be reiterated here. There may be unwanted side-effects because receptors for adrenalin are found at many other sites.

● Name a few other organs that respond to adrenalin.

● Adrenalin is the neurotransmitter used by the sympathetic nervous system so smooth muscle in organs of the digestive, respiratory, vascular and reproductive systems will all be affected.

● In the light of the previous answer, why do you think beta-blockers are used to treat anxiety disorder and panic?

● In anxiety disorders, perceptions of worry and panic about something that is worrying, but not catastrophically so, often spiral out of control in a kind of loop, where the person becomes worried, then worried about how worried they are, then worried at the magnitude of their worry response, and so on. Beta-blockers interrupt this loop by ensuring that the perception of worry does not have its usual self-fuelling effects on the body. It is only a short-term solution, since it does not address the causes of this thinking style.

To summarize, then, there is evidence that brain activity, and particularly the formation of memory, is facilitated by a small dose of stress. Adrenalin and blood glucose appear to be important in this linkage, for, if the effects of adrenalin are reversed, the effect disappears.

Case Report 3.1   Panic attack

Shirley is a 43-year-old woman who was brought into the Accident and
Emergency Unit by emergency ambulance after experiencing a panic attack
in a local supermarket. The paramedics reported that the call had come
through to control, describing a person who had collapsed and had chest pain.
When they arrived at the supermarket they found that Shirley was
hyperventilating (breathing very rapidly), complaining of dizziness, and chest
pain. She was sweating and shaking, and had a 'pins and needles' sensation in
her hands and feet. She was clearly terrified and said she 'thought she was
going to die'. The paramedics documented her pulse rate as being 120 bpm
and her respiratory rate as being 42. Her oxygen saturations were 100%. Her
blood pressure, taken in the ambulance, was 140/85 mmHg. They tried to
calm her down, and encourage her to relax and to rebreathe her expired air
from a paper bag. Although Shirley's symptoms reduced, she was still
hyperventilating and feeling dizzy. She told the ambulance crew that she has
had these attacks before and has been treated for anxiety.

In A&E, Shirley was thoroughly assessed, and the diagnosis of a panic attack
was confirmed. A nurse stayed with her, and talked her through breathing in
and out of the paper bag slowly, and gradually her 'pins and needles'
sensation resolved. Shirley was tearful, and told the nurse that it was the
anniversary of her mother's death later that week and that she always 'gets
worse' at this time of year. She also explained that she has 'battled' with
agoraphobia for a number of years. Recently her pet dog died and she has
since been finding it harder and harder to go out. At Shirley's request, her
husband was phoned and he arrived at the hospital. He told the staff that
Shirley's problems with anxiety were long-standing and she had been cared
for by the community mental health team in the past but was not seeing the
community mental health nurse (CMHN) presently.

The A&E doctor discussed how Shirley might benefit from seeing the CMHN
again, and that they could work with her to help her manage her anxiety.
Shirley agreed to be referred, and it was arranged for her to be visited by the
CMHN later that week. At this first visit, the nurse spent some time with
Shirley carrying out an assessment, and looking at what she saw as her
current problems. Shirley completed an anxiety rating scale scoring how she
feels before she goes out. The nurse asked Shirley to describe what she was
thinking when she was experiencing panic in a crowded place. These thoughts
included, 'I will make a fool of myself', 'I will be sick everywhere',
'Everybody will look at me with contempt', and 'I will embarrass my husband
and children'. These fears were then discussed and challenged. The nurse
and Shirley met every week, initially in her own home, and later in the
shopping centre. Shirley was encouraged to complete a thought diary and
together the nurse and Shirley developed a programme to help her gradually
face the situations she feared. The nurse also taught Shirley relaxation
techniques to use prior to going out. After two months, Shirley was able to go
round the supermarket alone without undue distress.

3.3.6 What use is stress?

● Look back over the effects of the stress response described in Sections 3.3.1–3.3.5. Summarize the main immediate effects of stress for yourself.

● The main components of the stress response would seem to be:
  - increasing the rate of circulation of the blood;
  - enriching the blood with energy-filled glucose and fatty acids from the body's stores;
  - stopping digestion;
  - stopping reproductive activity;
  - blunting sensitivity to pain;
  - getting the immune system ready to respond to pathogens;
  - making the mind alert and ready to learn.

In the rest of this section we will consider what use such responses are, and why they have been maintained in so many species of animals through evolutionary history.

Stress pioneers like Walter Cannon spoke of the stress response as an adaptation of the body to current conditions. Cannon said that stress got you ready for 'fight or flight'. What he meant was that animals (including humans) from time to time find themselves in extremely serious situations where their well-being or even survival is threatened.

A classic example of a serious situation would be a deer being pursued by a pack of wolves. The deer has to escape or fend off the wolves, or it will die. Describe how it might achieve this by outlining the sequence of events that occur as the deer is hunted, from its first awareness of the wolves' presence to the end of the chase. Describe the stress responses occurring at each stage of the hunt and explain the physiological background to each response. Indicate what use each response has for the deer's survival.

You might like to consider the deer's need for the maximum supply of blood possible to its muscles for running away, and its need for every reserve of energy supply that it has available. It will need to be alert, and to learn quickly what strategies are successful. It will need its immune cells ready in case it is wounded. It will need to blunt pain because it has to run even to the point of exhaustion and beyond.

This raises the obvious question: why doesn't the deer have these stress responses activated all the time? Surely it would be better to always be vigilant, since you never know when wolves are going to turn up? The problem with this solution is that everything in physiology comes with costs. The organism's energy is finite; making glucose available from storage means depleting the energy reserves. An animal running at that level all the time would need a lot of food to keep it going. And other processes that take up energy have to be shut off to keep up the maximum readiness. Digestive activity is halted. This makes sense in the short term – digestion requires energy, and there is no point expending energy on breaking down grass in the stomach, when by the time the nutrients from that grass become available for use, the animal will be in pieces inside a wolf. Similarly with reproduction – there is no point in keeping reproductive hormones circulating when the deer is going to be wolf-meat long before it could bring an offspring to term.

However, in the long term, animals have to digest or they will not survive and if they do not reproduce the species becomes extinct. The stress response is therefore a temporary switching of resources between long-term goals like reproduction, digestion, growth and tissue repair, and short-term goals like getting away from a dangerous situation alive. Eminent stress physiologist Robert Sapolsky (Sapolsky, 1998) likens the situation to investment. You will ultimately get more return on your money if you put it into a long-term investment account where the interest rate is high, but you cannot withdraw it quickly. However, there is no point in doing this if you don't have enough money to pay for food today. If you were behaving rationally, you would switch your financial planning according to the circumstances. First you would make sure you had enough available for day to day use. Then you might start to lock away any surplus. But if you had a financial crisis, you would want to make your money available for immediate use. The stress response does the physiological equivalent of this.

Summary of Section 3.3

1 The stress response involves signalling by the sympathetic nervous system, which releases adrenalin and noradrenalin, and by the hypothalamic-pituitary-adrenal axis, which effects cortisol release.

2 The stress response involves increases in heart rate and blood pressure, and decreases in digestive activity and reproductive hormone release.

3 Glucose and fatty acids are released into the circulation during a stress response.

4 Immune activity may be transiently stimulated by stress hormones, whilst sensitivity to pain can be reduced due to endorphin release.

5 The immediate response to stress is to enhance alertness and memory formation, through the effects of adrenalin and increased blood glucose.

6 The stress response seems to be an effective method for coping with a short-term crisis.

3.4 The costs of stress

The material we have covered so far seems paradoxical. In the first section, we noted the poorer health outcomes of low-grade civil servants, and suggested that these might well be to do with stress. In that context, stress would seem to be damaging and pathological. In the second and third sections, we reviewed the physiology of stress, and saw how it appears to be an adaptive, beneficial response that prepares the body to deal effectively with challenges. How can both these things be true?

To begin to answer this question, we need to distinguish between the short-term and the long-term consequences of the stress response. In the previous section, we considered only the immediate consequences of stress. What happens if the response persists?

3.4.1 The immune system

We begin with the immune system, since it is a common feeling that when we are stressed we are more likely to get a cold or 'flu. A number of studies have demonstrated this result. For example, John Jemmott and his colleagues at Princeton University studied dental students through the academic year (Jemmott et al., 1983). They measured the levels of IgA (type A immunoglobulin) in the students' saliva at five different times during the academic year.

● Look back at Book 3, Section 4.7.1. What is IgA?

◐ Immunoglobulins are proteins produced by the immune system, which play a part in the protection of the body from infection. There are five major types, including IgA.

The first measurement point was at the end of the summer, when the students had just returned from summer break. Levels of self-rated stress were low at this point. Then there were three measurements during the year. Finally, a fifth measurement was taken when the year's programme was complete and the students were going off for the next summer break. The results are shown in Figure 3.7. As you can see, the production of IgA was highest before and after the summer break, around 0.19–0.20 mg IgA secreted min^{-1}.

● Describe what happens for the rest of the year.

◐ There was a substantial drop in IgA production by November to about 0.18 mg min^{-1} but the lowest levels, around 0.17 mg min^{-1}, were recorded in April. By June, levels had risen and were slightly higher than they were in November.

● Do you think student examinations were held in May or June?

◐ We can surmise that April is the most stressful time of the year for these students and that their exams are held in May rather than June.

Figure 3.7 IgA secretion rates in dental students through the academic year.

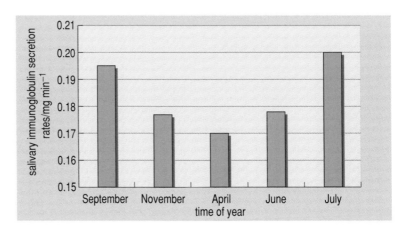

This study is very interesting, but as a demonstration that stress makes people vulnerable to infectious disease, it suffers from a number of limitations.

● Can you think of what some of the limitations of the study are?

● First, the study did not actually show that the participants got ill more often at stressful times, merely that their levels of one type of immunoglobulin were lower. Second, the study could not show that the stress of the academic year was causing the reduction. It could just be that people secrete less immunoglobulin in the winter when it is colder, or for some other reason, possibly related to daylength.

The dental student study was what is known as a naturalistic or observational design. That is to say, the students were doing what they would naturally be doing, and the researchers simply observed their responses. The problem with naturalistic designs is that often it is not possible to control all the factors that might be affecting your results (such as seasonality). In contrast to naturalistic designs, *experimental* designs are often better at demonstrating cause and effect. In an experimental design, you artificially create the situation in which you are interested, whilst keeping all other factors constant.

● Can you think of an experiment that you would do to investigate the effects of stress on susceptibility to infectious disease? What problems would there be in carrying out such an experiment?

● You might have recollected the experiment that examined wound healing in carers and non-carers described in Book 1, Section 2.12 (Kiecolt-Glaser et al., 1995) and used that to inform your design. Almost certainly you will have considered the ethical issues surrounding any experimental design that allows infectious disease susceptibility to increase, possibly without the participants knowing. Assessing health indicators, e.g. scoring stress levels accurately and measuring susceptibility to infection, may be difficult to do objectively and it would be difficult to adjust for the wide range of variables influencing the experimental outcomes.

One experiment that was conducted in this area to investigate such a problem is described below but you may have thought of an equally good design.

In this well-known study (Cohen et al., 1991), 394 healthy volunteers spend nine days at a research facility in Salisbury, England. (What on earth they did for nine days is not clear, but it was part of the controlled conditions of the experiment that they could not leave.) On arrival at the centre, they filled in questionnaires about their then current level of perceived stress, which gave them a current stress score on a scale of 0–12. The eager participants were then given nasal sprays containing the viruses that cause the common cold. For the next seven days, doctors monitored whether the participants had become infected with a virus, and also whether they showed the symptoms of colds.

Figure 3.8 shows the percentage of the participants developing a cold for each of the different levels of score on the stress index at the beginning of the experiment.

● What is the relationship between developing a cold and self-rated stress?

● The figure shows a strong positive correlation between stress at the beginning of the experiment and the outcome; the more stressed individuals were at the beginning, the more likely they were to end up with a cold. 47% of the most stressed individuals developed a cold, in contrast to 27% of the least stressed.

Since all participants were equally exposed to the cold viruses, the explanatory principle must be that the people who were more stressed were less able to fight off infection from the pathogen to which they had been exposed.

● Does this accord with the findings of Kiecolt-Glaser et al. (Book 1, Section 2.12)?

● Yes. In that study the experimental group members were all caring for dependants who had Alzheimer's disease and they tended to heal more slowly than the group members with no caring responsibilities. They also had reduced levels of interleukin-1; a measure of the efficacy of white cell metabolism (its role was described in Book 1, Section 2.12).

Figure 3.8 Percentage of participants developing a cold after exposure to a virus, plotted against their level of self-rated stress before the experiment began.

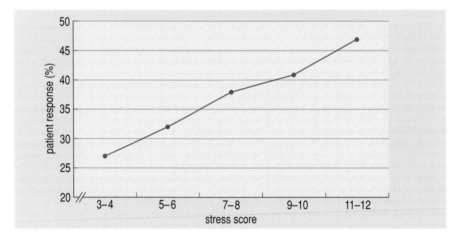

● How do you square the results of the Cohen et al. study with the evidence from Section 3.3.4 and Figure 3.6 that a dose of stress hormone actually *facilitates* the functioning of the immune system?

● The key to this puzzle is in Figure 3.6. The figure shows that whilst a small dose of corticosterone enhances immune functioning, a very large dose reduces it very severely. High or prolonged stress generates enough stress hormones to push the levels into that part of the response range where more hormone means less immune activity.

This, then, is the current consensus on stress hormones and immune functioning: the stress response provides a small transient activation of immune functioning, but then, as stress hormones build up, a reduction in immune functioning occurs, so that with severe or prolonged stress, the person is left at heightened risk of infectious disease. This mechanism seems able to explain a number of public health findings, such as the heightened risk of infections amongst those who are recently bereaved, going through life changes, isolated, or upset in other ways.

The stress hormones also have an inhibitory effect on a related set of bodily defences – inflammation. Inflammation is the tissue's response to local damage. It involves the tissue swelling up as fluids, which help in the defence and repair process, aggregate at the site. Cortisol and related substances, when applied in large doses, inhibit the inflammatory response. For this reason, they are often used as anti-inflammatory medicine. You might have come across cortisone or hydrocortisone cream as a treatment for a swelling. With these drugs, you are using the suppressive function of stress hormones to damp down your body's response.

This principle is also employed in some other drug treatments. There is a class of conditions (first introduced in Book 1, Section 3.7.2) called autoimmune disease where the immune system attacks the body's own tissues. Autoimmune diseases include some forms of rheumatism, inflammatory bowel disease, Graves' disease (Book 2, Case Report 3.1), and lupus. Cortisol-like hormones have sometimes been used to treat some autoimmune conditions, precisely because they damp down the activity of the immune system.

● Why do you think that treatment for autoimmune disease using cortisol-like hormones might be dangerous?

● For two reasons. One is that, with the immune system suppressed, the person could be vulnerable to infection. The second is that stress hormones have many negative consequences above and beyond their effect on the immune system, as was indicated in the case report on Crohn's disease (Book 1, Section 4.4).

In the next few sections we shall examine some of the negative consequences of chronic stress.

3.4.2 The cardiovascular system

We have seen that the short-term effect of the stress response is to increase the rate of blood circulation by increasing the pumping rate of the heart and constricting blood vessels. In the long term, however, stress is associated with heart disease. This is as true for rats and mice subjected to overcrowding as it is for low-grade civil servants experiencing work stress.

Basically, problems accumulate because higher blood pressure, if experienced frequently or constantly, causes greater wear and tear on blood vessels. Small tears or scars develop in the inner layer of the vessels. Once these imperfections have formed, fatty acids, circulating cells and other substances adhere to them, gradually causing obstructions. These obstructions are known as atherosclerotic plaques (Book 3, Section 2.6.1). Atherosclerotic plaques can stop the blood getting through to key tissues. Where they develop in the arteries that provide oxygenated blood to the heart itself, angina and heart attack can be the result. People with high stress levels also have more circulating fatty acids, which may exacerbate the growth of plaques.

● Why would people with high stress levels tend to have high levels of blood fatty acids?

● Because the cortisol response causes fatty acids to be released from fat cells, in order to provide energy (Section 3.3.3).

Plaque formation illustrates perfectly the trade-off between long-term and short-term efficiency in physiological systems. From a short-term point of view, if the environment is dangerous, then you need to have blood pumping at the maximum possible rate in case you need to do something dramatic. However, maintaining this rate will exhaust the system in the very long term. The best thing to do from the animal's point of view varies with the situation. If you are about to be eaten, there is simply no point in maintaining your arteries in good long term condition, since you will not live to reap the benefit. However, once you are safe for the immediate future, you should shift blood pressure down. The stress response is exquisitely designed to do this, but if it is activated too often, the cost is high.

3.4.3 Digestion

One of the most consistent findings in stress medicine research was that stress caused ulcers in the stomach, both in humans and non-human animals. Imagine everyone's surprise then, when in the 1980s, Australian researchers showed that ulcers were caused by a bacterium, *Helicobacter pylori* (Figure 3.9; see also Section 4.3.4 in Book 1). The discovery of *H. pylori* was a surprise for many reasons. The stomach is highly acidic, and no-one had thought that any bacteria could live there (*H. pylori* has a highly specialized structure that allows it to do so).

● How does *H. pylori* resist the hydrochloric acid in the stomach?

◔ *H. pylori* adheres to the mucosa, beneath the protective layer of mucus.

Moreover, literally dozens of studies showed increases in the incidence of ulcers in animals that were experimentally stressed, or in humans living through natural stress. For example, during the Blitz of 1940–1941, when residential areas of London were repeatedly bombed, there was a rise in the incidence of stomach ulcers amongst the population. So resistant was the establishment to the idea of an infectious cause for ulcers that one of the Australian researchers, Barry Marshall, had no choice but to infect himself with the bacteria; he experienced stomach inflammation as a result, thus proving that his account was basically correct.

Figure 3.9 Coloured scanning electron micrograph of *Helicobacter pylori* (yellow) on the lining of the stomach. Magnification × 4000.

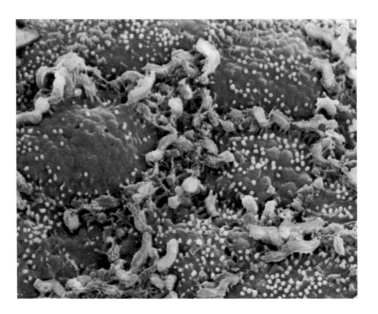

● If ulcers are caused by *H. pylori*, they cannot be caused by stress. Is this correct?

● No. Stress and the presence of the bacteria could interact to lead to ulcers. In particular, stress could reduce a person's resistance to the effects of the bacteria, just as in the immune system case.

It is now clear that there is an interaction between stress and the bacteria. Many people carry *H. pylori* in their stomachs, but most of them do not get ulcers. The difference between those who do and those who do not appears to be related to stress. In experimental animals, eliminating bacteria with antibiotic treatment makes stressor exposure less likely to lead to ulcers, and infection with bacteria potentiates the ulcer–stress link.

● What is a stomach ulcer?

● Ulcers are sores on the wall of the digestive tract (see Book 1, Figure 4.18). Stomach ulcers develop in areas where the stomach epithelium has been eroded.

● How is the stomach epithelium normally protected from erosion and why is erosion a particular risk?

● The walls are lined with a protective mucous membrane that is needed as protection against abrasive particles and the acidic stomach environment.

● How does *H. pylori* bring about inflammation of the gut?

● It produces toxins that damage the epithelial cells (i.e. the bacteria attack the mucous membrane).

During stress, stomach activity in general is suppressed. Secretion of digestive acid is reduced, and blood flow to the walls of the stomach is also lessened. In response to these changes, epithelial cell replacement slows down (recall that these cells are normally replaced on a five-day cycle; Book 1, Section 4.2.1) and the mucous membrane becomes thinner or more susceptible to damage, thereby giving the bacteria the opportunity to perforate it. An ulcer occurs when the protective layer is perforated, allowing stomach acids to begin attacking the walls of the stomach itself. There is some evidence that the risk of ulceration is higher when severe stress abates. With the reduction in stress, the stomach begins to produce acid again, but in the meantime the protective coating has been compromised and the acid damages the stomach wall itself.

3.4.4 Reproduction

As we have learnt in Section 3.3.4, another effect of a stressor was to reduce the production of reproductive hormones such as testosterone, oestrogen and progesterone. We would predict that such changes would disrupt sexual and reproductive behaviour.

In experimental animals, we know that this can happen. For example, one group of researchers exposed male rats to different kinds of stressors and then presented them with a mate (Retana-Marquez et al., 2003). Figure 3.10 shows the levels of

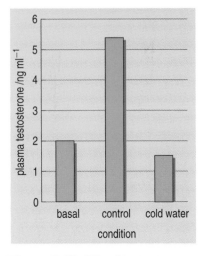

Figure 3.10 Blood testosterone levels in male rats under a baseline condition, exposed to a female rat (the control column), and exposed to a female rat after exposure to a cold water stressor.

blood testosterone in three groups of rats at one point in time early in the study: a baseline group of rats who had not been presented with a mate, a control group who had been presented with a mate, and a group of rats presented with a mate after exposure to a cold water stressor.

● Describe and interpret the data in Figure 3.10.

● Blood testosterone levels increase dramatically to 5.2 ng ml^{-1} in male rats exposed to females but fall below basal levels in rats that are shocked by contact with cold water prior to female exposure. Thus, presentation of a mate raises testosterone levels in unstressed rats but prior exposure to a stressful event abolishes this increase, and testosterone levels plummet to 1.5 ng ml^{-1}.

Since testosterone mediates sexual behaviour in the male, one would predict that the mating behaviour of the stressed rats would be disrupted. This is indeed what happened. The stressed group took longer to mount and inseminate the female rat than the controls.

● What implications might such findings have for human males?

● You would expect that stress might lead to loss of sexual desire, and disruptions of sexual performance.

In fact, transient sexual problems are quite common in the human male. The most common types are erectile dysfunction (impotence) and premature ejaculation. Both of these are associated with stress. Incidentally, they might appear to be opposite phenomena (one caused by an insufficient sexual response, the other caused by too much), but this is not the case. It turns out that erection is controlled by the parasympathetic branch of the autonomic nervous system, and so will require a calm and relaxed state to function optimally. Ejaculation is controlled by the sympathetic branch, and so will tend to be facilitated when that branch is highly activated. Since sympathetic and parasympathetic activities tend to be inversely related, this means that erectile dysfunction and premature ejaculation can often go together.

(As an aside, you might have heard that in Victorian Britain young men were advised to take a cold shower to take their minds off matters carnal!)

What about female sexual and reproductive behaviour in relation to stress? Sexual desire is often reduced by periods of stress, just as for males. Again, this can be demonstrated with animal models as well as clinical observation. Stress can also interfere with the monthly cycle of menstruation and ovulation. Cycles become longer and less regular, essentially because the hormonal signposts that guide the cycle (changing levels of oestrogen and progesterone) are less clear. In extreme cases, cycling shuts down altogether. This effect, known as **amenorrhea**, is commonly observed in women who are doing extreme amounts of physical exercise, such as athletes and dancers, and in anorexic patients, who induce extreme stress by eating insufficient amounts.

3.4.5 Brain structure and function

We saw in Section 3.3.5 that the short-term effect of the stress response is to enhance brain activity and memory formation. However, once again, the long-term effect of sustained stress is very different from the immediate effect of a single burst.

Much of the initial evidence in this area, as others in stress research, came from animal studies. Researchers showed that repeated stress eventually resulted in neurons in an area of the brain known as the hippocampus losing some of their dendrites (to locate the hippocampus in the brain, you can refer back to Book 2, Figure 1.9). For example, Magarinos et al. (1996) studied the tree shrew *Tupaia belangeri*. Two males were placed in cages separated by a wire mesh. Once a day, the mesh was removed, resulting in a competition between the males for dominance of the space. When this procedure was repeated day after day, there was a consistent winner and a consistent loser. The dominant individual would occupy the whole space, whilst the subordinate would avoid the dominant and stick to the periphery of the cage.

The researchers found that the cortisol levels of the subordinates (but not dominants) were greatly increased relative to the period before the study. After 28 days of interactions, the animals were sacrificed, and neurons in their hippocampi stained and measured. The researchers found that in the subordinate animals, which had had high stress levels for 28 days, the neurons had fewer dendritic branches and a reduction in the overall length of dendrites (Figure 3.11), than in control animals. Other studies have shown that exactly the same effect can be achieved by giving high doses of corticosterone, thus showing conclusively that it is the stress hormone that is responsible for the effect.

Why is this finding important? The hippocampus is located within the temporal lobe (Book 2, Figure 1.8) and is part of the limbic system that deals with emotional information in the brain. It has been found to be crucial in the formation and storage of memories. For example, damage to the hippocampus is often associated with memory loss or the inability to form new memories. The hippocampus consists of a web of interconnected neurons, and the encoding of information is via their interconnections. A loss of connections in the hippocampus can only be detrimental to memory function. The prediction would therefore be that sustained stress should cause memory impairment. This has been shown to be the case in experimental animals. When rats are stressed repeatedly, not only do hippocampal neurons lose connections, but the animals show impaired function in some tasks where they have to remember a location or a response.

It is naturally of the greatest interest to determine whether these findings transfer to humans, but ethically and practically this is a difficult topic to study. It has been known for some time that people with **post traumatic stress disorder**, for example, as a result of having served in the Vietnam war, perform less well than matched controls on a task where they have to remember a list of words for a short period of time. In addition, adults who were psychologically abused as children have similar memory problems.

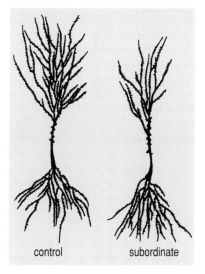

control   subordinate

Figure 3.11 Representative neurons from the hippocampus of (a) control tree shrew; (b) subordinate tree shrew after social stress. (Golgi stain; magnification approximately × 400)

Though it is not possible to look at the connections of individual neurons in living human beings, it has recently become possible to examine the structure of the living brain in some detail using magnetic resonance imaging (MRI) to create a detailed image of the brain's structure. J. Douglas Bremner and colleagues (Bremner et al., 1997) used MRI to show that the left hippocampus in adults who had been sexually or physically abused as children was on average 12% smaller than in control subjects. This would presumably account for the observed memory deficits in such groups.

We know that axons can regrow. In fact, decades of scientific orthodoxy maintaining that the brain cannot grow new neurons have recently been shown to be wrong. Cessation of stress for a few weeks leads to a return to structural normality for hippocampal neurons in the rat. This suggests that the effects of stress on the brain, though serious, are not always irreversible.

Summary of Section 3.4

1   Long-term stress reduces immune system functioning and increases susceptibility to infectious disease.

2   Long-term stress increases the risk of heart disease by hastening the formation of atherosclerotic plaques.

3   Long-term stress is associated with stomach ulcers, through an interaction between stress-induced physiological changes and the bacterium *Helicobacter pylori.*

4   Extreme stress suppresses reproductive function in humans and non-human animals.

5   Severe stress has been associated with loss of neural connections in the hippocampus, and associated loss of memory function.

3.5 Mediators of stress

We will now consider the factors that make life more or less stressful. We have seen that the stress response can be elicited by a very wide array of different situations. What is it that they all have in common? To answer this question, we will consider first animal and then human studies.

3.5.1 Non-human animal studies

In principle, any change in the environment that could be associated with danger can elicit the stress response. In animals that are normally solitary, it could be placement with other individuals. In animals that normally live in a colony, it could be isolation. Exposure to a predator such as a cat, or even just placement in a new habitat with no cover, is enough to elicit a stress response in a rat or mouse.

A number of studies have shown that the ability to control the stressor is of fundamental importance in mediating the stress response. The classic way of demonstrating this is a paradigm in which one animal is 'yoked' to another. (They are actually in separate cages and are only metaphorically yoked together, in the sense that whatever happens to the one happens to the other.) For example, animal A receives an unpleasant noise, and can turn it off by pressing a lever or running on a wheel. Animal B is subjected to the same noise when animal A receives it, for the same length of time, and at the same intensity. Thus both animals receive precisely the same timing and intensity of stressor.

In a yoked experiment, since both animals receive the same stressor, you might think they will show the same stress response, but they don't.

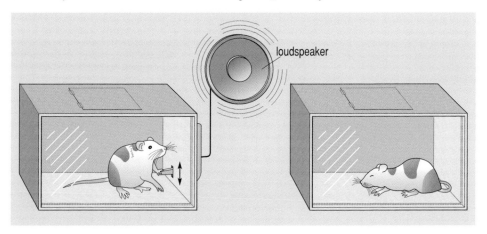

Figure 3.12   A yoked animal experimental set-up.

In fact, the animal that can control the stressor shows a much reduced stress response. The most likely explanation for this is that simply performing the behaviour truncates the response. After all, once the animal has done whatever it needs to do to turn the noise off, there is no further need to be stressed. For the passive animal, on the other hand, it never knows when the noise will terminate or what it can do to escape.

Similar experiments have shown that lack of predictability is also an important stress mediator. If a stressor is reliably preceded by a warning light, the stress response is reduced, even though the animal still gets the stressor at the same duration and intensity. In fact, there is little it can do to prepare itself for the stressor but in all probability the existence of a warning light means that the animal does not have to be in a state of preparedness all the time, but can feel safe when the light is not on.

Finally, if animals have outlets for frustration, whether in the form of a lever to press, a bar to chew, or a subordinate to attack, the stress response is also reduced relative to that for having no such outlet.

● What implications might these animal findings have for human stress management?

● They suggest that people can reduce their stress levels by finding ways of predicting stressors, feeling in control of them, or taking out their frustration in other ways. These principles are indeed used in stress management (see next section).

Control and outlets for frustration combine in an interesting way in social animals whose groups have a hierarchy or rank system. Baboons, for example, live in large social groups within which there are clear differentials of rank (Figure 3.13). High-ranking animals are more likely to mate, and can take food from lower ranking ones. High-ranking individuals tend to be more physically powerful than low-ranking ones, and demonstrate this frequently but sporadically by attacking those lower down the hierarchy. The highest ranking individuals, of course, have no-one to attack them, save for the rare occasions when there is a challenge to their dominance.

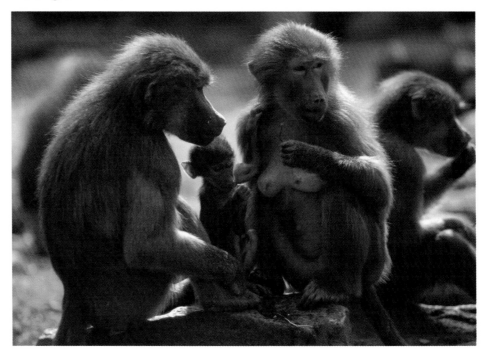

Figure 3.13 A baboon social group.

In baboons, low-ranking individuals have raised cortisol levels and evidence of stress-related health problems. It is easy to see how the principles of predictability, control and outlets for frustration apply. Subordinates get attacked by dominants. They never know when this will happen and there is nothing they can do to control it, since they are not physically capable of stopping it (they would not be subordinate otherwise). They cannot leave, since baboons, amongst the most social of monkeys, can only really survive as members of large groups. Middle-ranking individuals can at least displace their frustration by attacking someone lower-ranking than them after they are attacked by a dominant. Individuals at the very bottom of the hierarchy do not have even this option.

It turns out that it is not universally true that high-ranking individuals have lower stress hormones levels than low-ranking ones. In monkeys such as tamarins (*Saguinus oedipus*) that live in small, family-based groups with just a breeding pair, their offspring, and a few young cousins who are acting as breeding helpers, there are no hierarchical differences in cortisol levels. And even in baboons and other rank-based groups, when the hierarchy is unstable or the dominant is being frequently challenged for top position, the dominant's cortisol levels rise just as high as everyone else's. From the point of view of stress, it seems that dominants want to avoid instability, and from the subordinate's point of view, it would probably be better if they could avoid the rank system altogether and live in a small family group somewhere. Doesn't this bring to mind the civil service example with which we began the chapter?

Finally, it is worth noting that there are considerable differences between individuals in the stress response. In monkeys, for example, it is possible to identify individuals known as 'hot reactors', whose cortisol response to a given stressor is relatively large, and persists for a long time, compared to the response in other individuals. The monkeys that are hot reactors in one experiment will also be hot reactors in a subsequent one, suggesting that the response to stress is partly set by enduring aspects of our temperament.

3.5.2 Human studies

The three principles of control, predictability and outlets for frustration transfer very easily from non-human animals to humans. The classic 'yoked' experiments have also been performed with human participants. The person is subjected to a loud unpleasant noise, which they can turn off by pressing a key or some other action. The passive individual just has to endure it until it stops. All the hallmarks of the stress response are greater in the passive individual.

The same kind of design can be used to study the effects of predictability. A light warning of the imminence of an unpleasant noise does indeed make it less stressful than an unpredictable noise. In the London Blitz, the biggest rises in the incidence of peptic ulcers were seen not in the centre of the city, but in the suburbs. The centre of the city was bombed every night, whereas a particular suburb might or might not be bombed. People living in the city centre could not control the bombing, of course, but at least they could predict that it was going to happen. People living in the suburbs, presumably, were constantly unsure whether they were going to have to rush for the shelters or not.

Across all developed societies that have so far been studied, there are socio-economic gradients in health, with those at the top of the social hierarchy having longer life and better health outcomes than those at the bottom. This applies to a wide range of illnesses, from infectious disease to heart disease. Interestingly, these gradients persist in very wealthy contemporary societies, where even the poorest people are above the absolute poverty line, and in societies where access to health care is universal and free. The best explanation in these contexts is that life is more stressful for those lower down the socio-economic hierarchy. Such people have less control over what they do; when and where they do it; they are probably more subject to unpredictable change; and their lower incomes may give them fewer alternative outlets for frustration. This is probably the best explanation of the Whitehall data with which we began this chapter. The people in the low grades may have less responsibility, but they also have much less control over what they have to do, compared to, say, a head of department. This appears to be linked to greater stress and all the health consequences that go with it.

Case Report 3.2 Work-related stress

Amanda is a 47-year-old woman who presented at her GP surgery complaining of exhaustion, sleepless nights, headaches and indigestion. During the ensuing discussion with her GP it became clear that, despite a relatively stress-free home life, Amanda was experiencing work-related stress as a result of restructuring activities at her workplace and was finding it difficult to face going into work at all. As the restructuring process had progressed, Amanda felt that her job role and responsibilities had been changed and devalued without appropriate consultation; a new layer of middle management had been appointed above her; and her role had been downgraded with a potential loss of earnings and career progression. Despite being actively involved in union and consultation groups, Amanda felt extremely frustrated that management was not listening to employees and that the working environment and roles were constantly changing in a very unpredictable manner as new phases of restructuring were rolled out. Taking up an offer of voluntary redundancy with a severance package had seemed one way of gaining some control over her future but after applying for the offer after weeks of very tough decision making, Amanda was told that she was not in the appropriate staff category to take advantage of the offer and was turned down. Increasing feelings of anger and distress at her lack of control over such events affected Amanda's ability to cope with situations generally. The stress began to affect her home life too – she found it increasingly difficult to carry out normal decision-making tasks and felt too exhausted to do anything but the most minor domestic duties. She woke most nights between 2.30 am and 4.00 am and was unable to get back to sleep after this time. Her interest in social activities had declined and she stopped making contact with friends and family. Her immediate family noticed her lack of communication and general air of despondence and persuaded her to make a GP appointment.

After considerable discussion, Amanda's GP ran a quick paper score stress assessment test on Amanda and concluded that she was suffering significant stress and was possibly on the verge of a major depression. She signed Amanda off work for a minimum period of three weeks, made another appointment to see her after one week and referred her for stress counselling. After further time away from work, Amanda began to develop a more positive outlook on life, renegotiated her employment contract and returned to full time employment.

It is clear from Case Report 3.2 that the effects of stress are not confined to the immediate stressful environment but can affect all aspects of an individual's life. The causes of stress, however, appear to be mediated through common routes.

● Think back to our discussion of stress mediators. What aspects of Amanda's work experience (Case Report 3.2) have probably contributed to her stress?

● Amanda has experienced lack of control, unpredictability of stressors and lack of an effective outlet for her frustration.

Another factor of particular importance for humans is social support. We are a quintessentially social species, and do not seem to fare at all well when isolated. Numerous studies have shown that married people, or people with close friends and family available, live longer, have a better immune response, recover more quickly from surgery, and have lower levels of cortisol than single people or people who lack a social network (Section 1.4 of this book).

● Do findings such as those described above mean that the lack of social support *causes* ill health?

● Not necessarily. Correlation is never sufficient to prove causation. It could be the case that people who are chronically ill have difficulty maintaining active social relationships and so end up isolated. Alternatively, it could be the case that some other factor (for example, having an anxious or hostile personality) makes individuals *both* socially isolated *and* vulnerable to ill health.

Concerns about causation are allayed to some extent by longitudinal studies in which individuals are followed to see if, when their level of social support changes, their level of stress-related ill health changes too. If it does, then it is likely that the effect is actually causal rather than just a correlation. Such studies have shown that when social support changes, the symptoms of stress tend to follow suit. For example, bereavement, separation and divorce are associated with reductions in immune functioning and an increased incidence of disease.

Just as there are hot reactor monkeys, who have elevated cortisol responses, there are human individuals who are especially prone to stress. One example is what is known as the **type A personality**. In the 1950s, two American cardiologists noted that many of their patients seemed to share the same personality patterns. In fact, according to one account, the original observation stemmed from the person whose job it was to re-upholster the chairs in the clinic waiting room. He noticed that the chairs were being quickly worn, but not uniformly – the waiting patients were ripping the fronts of the arms and the front of the seat. You could only do this if you were sitting, fidgety and impatient, literally on the edge of your seat. This pattern of wear was apparently only observed at the heart clinic, not in the waiting rooms of other kinds of patients. The doctors, Meyer Friedman and Roy Rosenman, noted that this chimed with their experience of heart patients, who were impatient, aggressive, fidgety, and always in a hurry. This was the origin of the type A personality concept. Friedman and Rosenman defined the type A personality as involving a constant sense of hurry or time urgency, a ceaseless striving after (often changing or undefined) goals, competitiveness and hostility. Subsequent research on the association between type A characteristics and heart disease has produced only mixed results, but there is general acceptance that this type of personality is associated with a particularly large stress response.

Fortunately, people can be counselled to reduce the impact of their type A behaviour. They can learn to manage anger, or to avoid the situations that make them stressed, and such counselling seems to be effective in helping them avoid heart problems, whilst not, as the competitive type As often fear, compromising their job performance.

3.5.3 Managing stress

Stress physiologist Robert Sapolsky has argued that although all mammals show the stress response, humans may be particularly prone to the negative effects of long-term or chronic stress. This is because we have the capacity to mentally anticipate and worry about potential problems well before they occur. In contrast, other species are not stressed by situations until they actually sense them physically. For example, a zebra will become stressed about lions if it sees, hears or smells one, but tends not to give lions much thought if there is no perceptual evidence that they are around. Human beings, on the other hand, can worry about the distant future, or things that could possibly happen, like an economic crash in a few years' time, or the collapse of pension plans. Once we start worrying about such things, it is easy to end up worrying about them all the time, since they are not likely to be resolved quickly, and they do not depend on any immediate factors or stimuli. We know that the stress response in humans can be evoked by the mere *thought* of a stressor. Thus there is a danger that, as probably the most cognitively sophisticated species on the planet, we end up as the most stressed one.

Lest this all seem too depressing, it is not clear that humans must always be more stressed than the lower order but happier beasts. For one thing, there are certain animal examples of chronic stress. Subordinate animals show the hallmarks of chronic stress, and rats become stressed every time they are put into a new environment, whether there is evidence of danger there or not. If you wanted to put this anthropomorphically, you could say that they worry about the possibility of danger, even though there is no actual evidence. In this sense they are being chronic worriers just like humans.

Above all though, the human cognitive capacities that can make us vulnerable to worry, can also liberate us from it. People can learn to adapt to even the most difficult situations simply by thinking about them more constructively. For example, you can reframe the situation to think about the advantages and the aspects of it that you can control. You can change your environment to make it more predictable (and ideally controllable too). You can develop hobbies as outlets for frustration and learn techniques such as yoga for relaxation. There is plenty of evidence that counselling in stress management is quite effective, and we have already seen how the impact of type A behaviour can be reduced by simple techniques. Stress is now recognized as a work-place hazard that is both predictable and preventable, and employers are required to carry out risk assessments to consider and address the issues of stress.

Overall, then, there is perhaps more room for optimism in humans than in other animals. The stress response is a powerful, double-edged sword, with short-term advantages and long-term costs. We can anticipate and control aspects of the environment enough to avoid some of the worst pitfalls, if we make the effort to do so.

Summary of Section 3.5

1   In humans and in other animals, key factors mediating the magnitude of stress are predictability, control, and outlets for frustration.

2   In many species with stable social hierarchies, subordinate animals are more stressed than dominant ones.

3   In human societies, there are socio-economic gradients in stress-related diseases, with more privileged social groups having better health and longer life.

4   Social support is also a key factor protecting people from stress-related disease.

5   There are differences between individuals in the reactivity of their stress systems. In particular, the personality type known as type A has been associated with the risk of heart disease.

6   Stress can be managed by psychological techniques that involve reframing the problem to emphasize aspects that can be controlled.

3.6 Conclusions

The human body has been described as being controlled by three interconnected major systems. The nervous system receives information from the senses and initiates appropriate behaviour. The endocrine system orchestrates the different tissues of the body to maintain homeostasis and keep vital functions running. Finally, the immune system protects the body from foreign materials and infections. In this course, you have learned about all of these systems. This chapter, however, has suggested that they are all intimately interconnected. We see this in action in the stress response. The whole body needs to gear up or gear down its activity according to the immediate needs of the context. An emergency, perceived by the nervous system, requires action. The nervous system signals the endocrine system to provide us with extra oxygen and energy. This feeds back to the nervous system, making us more alert. The immune system is activated. Non-vital systems are shut down. The three systems act as one to prepare the organism for fight or flight.

This reaction cannot be without its costs, however. Stress also illustrates the way that health and disease have to be considered holistically. Your likelihood of succumbing to an infectious disease is not independent of your state of mind. Your likelihood of a heart attack is not independent of your hormones. The three great systems are linked through the stress response, and so what goes on in any one system can affect the healthy functioning of both of the others.

Questions for Chapter 3

Question 3.1 (LO 3.1)

Decide whether the following statements about the stress response are true or false.

(a) The sympathetic nervous system signals the adrenal glands to release cortisol.

(b) One effect of the stress response is to make additional blood glucose available by conversion of glycogen.

(c) You would expect prolonged stress to lead to the build up of fat deposits in the body.

(d) Endorphins are the body's natural equivalents of morphine.

(e) Adrenalin is released more quickly than cortisol in response to a stressor.

(f) Beta-blockers inhibit the effect of adrenalin on mind and body.

(g) Prolonged stress increases immunoglobulin levels in the saliva.

Question 3.2 (LOs 3.3, 3.4)

Fill in the table below outlining both the short-term and long-term effects of stress on different body systems.

System	Short-term	Long-term
circulation		
immune system		
brain		
reproductive system		

Question 3.3 (LOs 3.5, 3.6)

It has been suggested that people in lower occupational positions have poorer health because of greater stress.

(a) How would you test this hypothesis?

(b) What recommendations would you make for employers to improve the health of their lower-grade employees?

Question 3.4 (LO 3.7)

A great deal of the work on the stress system has involved experiments on non-human animals which are then taken as a model of the human stress response. Give one argument for and one argument against such research, on (a) scientific and (b) ethical grounds.

References

Bremner, J. D. et al. (1997) Magnetic resonance imaging-based measurement of hippocampal volume in posttraumatic stress disorder related to childhood physical and sexual abuse – a preliminary report. *Biological Psychiatry*, **41**, 23–32.

Cahill, L., Prins, B., Weber, M. and McGaugh, J. L. (1994) β-adrenergic activation and memory for emotional events. *Nature*, **371**, 702–704.

Cohen, S., Tyrell, D. A. J. and Smith, A. P. (1991) Psychological stress and susceptibility to the common cold. *New England Journal of Medicine*, **325**, 606–612.

Gold, P. E. (1986) Glucose modulation of memory storage processing. *Behavioural and Neural Biology*, **45**, 342–349.

Jemmott, J. B. et al. (1983) Academic stress, power motivation and decrease in secretion rate of salivary secretory immunoglobin A. *Lancet*, June, 1400–1402.

Kiecolt-Glaser, J. K., Marucha, P. T., Malarkey, W. B., Mercado, A. M. and Glaser, R. (1995) Slowing of wound healing by psychological stress. *Lancet*, **346**, 1194–1196.

Magariños, A. M., McEwen, B. S., Flugge, G. and Fuchs E. (1996) Chronic psychosocial stress causes apical dendritic atrophy of hippocampal CA3 pyramidal neurons in subordinate tree shrews. *Journal of Neuroscience*, **16**, 3534–3540.

Migneault, B. et al. (2004) The effect of music on the neurohormonal stress response to surgery under general anesthesia. *Anesthesia and Analgesia*, **98**, 527–532.

Retana-Marquez, S. et al. (2003) Changes in masculine sexual behaviour, corticosterone and testosterone in response to acute and chronic stress in male rats. *Hormones and Behavior*, **44**, 327–337.

Sapolsky, R. (1998) *Why Zebras Don't Get Ulcers: An Updated Guide to Stress, Stress-Related Diseases, and Coping*. New York: W. H. Freeman.

Wiegers, G. et al. (1993) Differential effects of corticosteroids on rat peripheral blood T-lymphocyte mitogenesis in vivo and in vitro. *American Journal of Physiology*, **265**, E825-E830.

A HEALTHY BABY

4.1 Introduction: the cycles of life

For any mammalian species, reproduction is a compelling yet hazardous aspect of life. For us, the ideal endpoint of reproduction is the delivery of a healthy baby, an overwhelming event that brings much happiness into our lives. So you may be asking why we have included reproduction in a book entitled *Life's Challenges*. One reason is that 'everything in physiology comes with costs'. Pregnancy is particularly costly for the mother as the developing fetus draws on maternal energy resources to fuel its growth and development. Another reason that may occur to you is that while the arrival of a new baby in the family is a wonderful event, this nevertheless disrupts the routines established within a household; babies do not have timetables for meals and sleeping! Employment and work patterns of the parents are affected because good baby care requires much time, possibly reducing income from employment, and expensive cots, prams and baby clothes need to be bought. A baby's need to be fed once or twice or more frequently at night, means that parents suffer lack of sleep, with consequent debilitating effects (Chapter 2). For mothers who do not have the support of a partner or family, the pressures of coping with the arrival of a new baby can sometimes be overwhelming. So while giving birth to a healthy baby and caring for the child bring immeasurable happiness and fulfilment, these experiences have considerable cost measured in terms of time and effort as well as money. The resulting stress may be difficult to cope with; recall the effects of stress that we examined in Chapter 3.

In this chapter our focus is on the cellular and physiological processes of reproduction, and on how these processes culminate in producing a healthy embryo, with the potential to develop into a healthy baby. We begin by examining the processes of **gametogenesis** (the production of gametes) and fertilization, and their hormonal control. In both men and women, gametogenesis is cyclic but in women the cycle is more complicated because there are the two components: **oogenesis**, production of eggs that are released (ovulated) at an arrested stage of meiosis (Section 1.2.3) and are called **oocytes**, and preparation of the uterus for pregnancy.

On average, men produce about 300–600 spermatozoa per gram of testis per second and around 500 million spermatozoa may be released in one ejaculate. In contrast one menstrual cycle produces just one, occasionally two, oocytes each month. Males invest their resources in producing huge quantities of tiny spermatozoa, with very little cytoplasm, each with a head about 5–7 µm long, and a tail 40–50 µm long (see Figure 4.4 later). Any one of these could fertilize an egg which would develop into another human life. In contrast, women invest much more resource into producing each oocyte as an oocyte is a large cell, with much cytoplasm, about 100 µm in diameter.

The mature oocyte is released into the uterus at around day 15 of the menstrual cycle and survives for about 5 days, so the time available each month for fertilization is quite short. It is estimated that worldwide, about 85–90% of couples achieve conception within 2 years of trying. For the 10% or more who are infertile (World Health Organization, 2004), infertility causes considerable stress and unhappiness, and much research effort has been spent on examining the causes of infertility. Techniques of *in vitro* fertilization (IVF) enable many couples who are having difficulty in conceiving, to achieve successful pregnancies with good outcomes. Undergoing a treatment cycle for IVF is a complex and challenging process, as we shall see in Sections 4.5 and 4.6.

Even after fertilization, there is no guarantee of a healthy embryo. We saw in Section 1.2.3 that a surprisingly high percentage of oocytes and sperm have harmful genetic or chromosomal mutations, so most fertilized eggs do not develop normally and are aborted spontaneously at a very early stage of pregnancy. Certain mutations are not severe enough to prevent development of a fetus to term (birth) and are manifested as heritable genetic diseases. However, the incidence of harmful mutations found in live births is relatively low.

In recent years there has been concern about the effects of environmental pollution on human fertility. Exposure to radiation and chemical pollution is hazardous for developing oocytes and spermatozoa. The developing embryo is also susceptible to damage from harmful substances such as drugs and alcohol consumed by the mother.

Although we have emphasized problems with infertility, genetic diseases, and effects of pollution on the fetus, most established pregnancies are successful and end in delivery of a healthy baby or babies! A healthy baby is the culmination of fetal development, a complex set of processes and stages that begins with the fertilization of an oocyte by a sperm cell. So we begin by examining gametogenesis, where we see the most complex degree of endocrine control in which three tiers of endocrine glands, the hypothalamic–pituitary axis and the gonads, interact in controlling multiple stages of complex cyclic processes (Book 2, Section 3.5).

Summary of Section 4.1

1   Producing a healthy baby is costly in terms of energy, cash and emotional resources and therefore may be regarded as one of the challenges of life.

2   The successful completion of gametogenesis and fertilization are both essential for conception.

3   There is a high incidence of chromosomal and genetic abnormalities in oocytes and sperm; a proportion of abnormalities may be related to environmental pollutants.

4   Although fertilization of the oocyte is a random event, around 85–90% of couples achieve conception within two years of trying.

5   Infertile couples may have the option of *in vitro* fertilization, which can achieve pregnancy and the birth of a healthy baby.

4.2 Spermatogenesis and the spermatogenic cycle

In Book 2, we saw how hormones secreted by the hypothalamus and anterior pituitary, two key endocrine glands, control the processes of life and maintain homeostasis by controlling the rates of secretion of other hormones. The hypothalamus plays the central role in controlling the functions of the testis which are: **spermatogenesis**, production of sperm, and secretion of sex steroids, mainly testosterone. In order to understand these processes we begin by examining the anatomical and functional organization of the testis, and the stages of spermatogenesis. We then move on to study the hormonal control of testicular function.

4.2.1 The male reproductive system and spermatogenesis

Development of the testis (Section 1.2.3) is initiated in male embryos during the sixth week of pregnancy when the *SRY* gene is expressed. The SRY protein initiates development of the testes, and suppresses development of the female reproductive system. The developing testes move out of the abdominal cavity and descend into the scrotum, a process completed by the 35th–40th week of pregnancy. Baby boys are born with relatively large testes, which secrete testosterone, but secretion declines from about 2 months after birth and blood testosterone levels remain low from 3–5 months until puberty. Throughout childhood, the male reproductive system grows slowly until puberty, at about 12–15 years of age, when there is a spurt of rapid growth and development.

The male reproductive system comprises a pair of testes, a prostate gland and a duct system that culminates in the penis (Figure 4.1). Spermatogenesis takes place in the testes, and the optimum temperature for sperm production is about 2–3 °C cooler than body temperature. The testes are suspended outside the body cavity in the scrotum, and if they do not descend from their original position close to the kidneys, spermatogenesis cannot occur because of the high temperature.

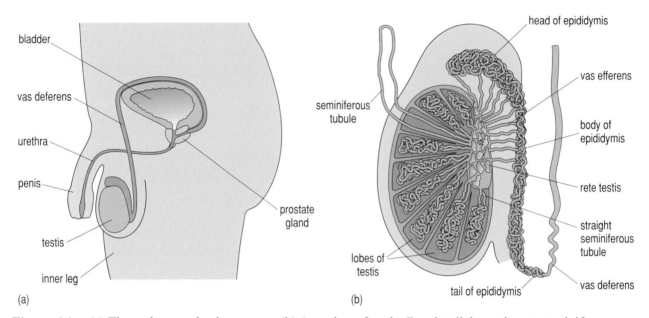

Figure 4.1 (a) The male reproductive system. (b) A section of testis. For simplicity, only one seminiferous tubule per lobe is shown; in reality there are many thousands. One of the tubules is shown extended.

Each testis is made up of large numbers of coiled **seminiferous tubules**, within which sperm production occurs. The seminiferous tubules end in a collecting area, from which a larger tube, the *vas efferens*, carries mature sperm into the **epididymis**. This is a collection of small tubules, in which the spermatozoa undergo maturation before entering the muscular walled **vas deferens**, which empties into the urethra at the base of the prostate (Figure 4.1).

In order to understand the functional organization of the testis, we need to move to the tissue and cellular levels of organization. Sperm production occurs inside the seminiferous tubules. Between the tubules there is interstitial tissue containing **Leydig cells**, which secrete sex steroids, mainly testosterone, and some oestrogen. So the two functions, production of sperm and secretion of sex steroids, are located in two compartments, the seminiferous tubules and the interstitial tissue, respectively (Figures 4.2 and 4.3). The two compartments are separated by a physical barrier, made up of two layers of fibrous basement membrane enclosing a tight-knit layer of cells, known as the **blood–testis barrier**. This barrier is of crucial importance for two reasons. First, sperm cannot penetrate the barrier and so do not leak into the systemic and lymphatic circulations. The immune system does not tolerate spermatozoa (i.e. sperm) and will produce antispermatozoal antibodies in response to spermatozoal antigens. Second, the barrier also prevents free passage of proteins, ions and sugars from the blood to the fluid inside the tubules, thereby providing a controlled chemical environment, optimal for spermatogenesis.

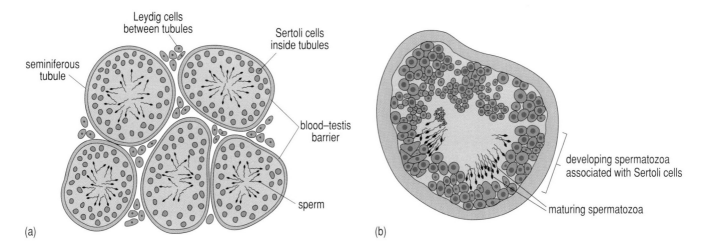

Figure 4.2 (a) Cross-section through a set of seminiferous tubules. The Leydig cells secrete testosterone. (b) Cross-section through a single seminiferous tubule showing 'wedges' of tubule at different stages of sperm production.

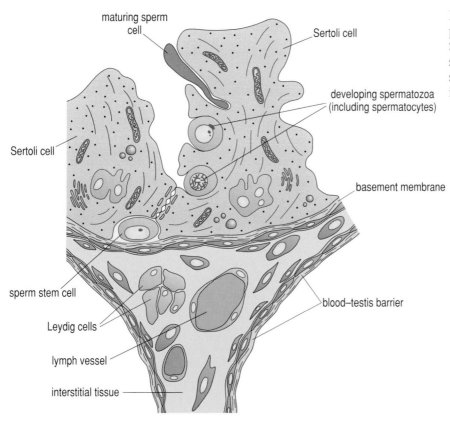

Figure 4.3 Cross-section through part of adult testicular tissue. Two Sertoli cells are shown, part of the seminiferous epithelium lining of a seminiferous tubule, and also some interstitial tissue containing Leydig cells.

Inside an active seminiferous tubule, spermatogenesis shows organization in time and space. The seminiferous tubules are lined with seminiferous epithelium, comprising specialized **Sertoli cells** within which are tucked diploid sperm stem cells (Figures 4.2 and 4.3). Proliferation of stem cells and the subsequent stages of spermatogenesis are supported paracrinally (locally), by testosterone and by its more potent derivative *dihydrotestosterone* (DHT), synthesized by the Sertoli cells.

● The blood–testis barrier prevents movement of substances such as proteins and sugars from interstitial tissue into the seminiferous tubules. How does testosterone secreted by Leydig cells in interstitial tissue gain access to Sertoli cells inside the tubules?

● Testosterone is a steroid, and it can therefore cross the lipid-rich cell membranes and the cytoplasm of the cells forming the blood–testis barrier.

Spermatozoa that are at various developmental stages and are tucked into the Sertoli cells gradually push their way towards the centre of the tubule (Figures 4.2 and 4.3). Sperm stem cells positioned at the base of Sertoli cells divide by mitosis and their daughter cells divide several times, producing groups of developing sperm cells, *spermatocytes*. Each *spermatocyte* undergoes meiosis, and the resulting daughter cells mature into spermatozoa (Figure 4.3).

● How many daughter cells are formed by meiosis from each spermatocyte? How do the daughter cells differ in terms of chromosome number from the stem cells and somatic cells in the body?

● Four daughter cells are formed from each spermatocyte that undergoes meiosis. Each of the four daughter cells has 23 chromosomes, a haploid number, in contrast with stem cells from which they derive which, like all somatic cells in the body, are diploid, having 46 chromosomes (Figure 1.4).

The daughter cells (developing sperm cells) mature and develop the typical head and tail structure of spermatozoa (Figure 4.4), with mitochondria concentrated at the base of the tail. The spermatozoa cannot swim and so fertilize an oocyte until they have passed through the epididymis, where they are bathed in nutritious sugary secretions, e.g. fructose, and coated with glycoproteins from the prostate gland. By the time sperm move into the vas deferens, they are capable of swimming in the female reproductive tract.

We began this chapter by stating that both spermatogenesis and oogenesis are cyclic. It is the initiation of spermatogenesis that is cyclic. One stem cell generates a related group of spermatozoa at a characteristic rate; it takes 64 days for completion of spermatogenesis, from mitosis in a stem cell to a group of haploid spermatozoa. Once spermatogenesis has been initiated at a particular location in a tubule, the stem cell there cannot initiate any new development for 16 days. In some way, a stem cell can 'measure' this period, the length of the **spermatogenic cycle**.

● What is the ratio of the time taken for completion of spermatogenesis to that taken for the spermatogenic cycle?

● The spermatogenic cycle lasts for 16 days; spermatogenesis takes 64 days. So the ratio is 1 : 4; the cycle length is one-quarter of the total time taken for completion of spermatogenesis.

● How many waves of spermatogenesis are taking place in a 'wedge' in a seminiferous tubule representing cells derived from one stem cell?

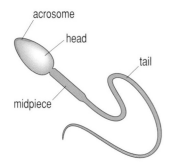

Figure 4.4 Structure of a mature human sperm. Head length is 5–7 μm, and tail length about 45 μm.

● Four successive waves of spermatogenesis must be taking place at the same time in a wedge of seminiferous tubule where groups of developing sperm are developing from a stem cell.

Along the length of a seminiferous tubule, there are groups of developing spermatozoa at different stages of development, e.g. a group in one part of the tubule will have four waves of spermatogenesis each initiated at a different time to those in groups further along the tube. A cross-section of a human seminiferous tubule contains wedges with groups having four waves of spermatogenesis at different stages to those in groups in adjacent wedges (Figure 4.2b).

● Why is it important for there to be groups of developing spermatozoa at different stages of development, rather than the development stages in all the tubules being synchronized?

● If all stem cells entered mitosis simultaneously, and all groups of developing sperm were at the same stage, there would be periodic pulses of release of huge numbers of spermatozoa with no sperm release in between times. This would cause long periods of male infertility. Initiation of mitosis in stem cells at staggered time intervals provides a constant supply of mature spermatozoa.

Spermatogenesis can only take place with appropriate hormonal support. In the next section we move on to consider the hormonal control of spermatogenesis.

4.2.2 Hormonal control of testicular function

In young boys, spermatogenesis does not occur, the testes are small, and blood testosterone levels are low, < 0.1 ng ml^{-1}. Spermatogenesis begins during puberty around the age of 14 years (age range is 12–15 years) and evidence from research indicates that increased pulsatile secretion of gonadotropin-releasing hormone (GnRH) by the hypothalamus initiates and drives puberty.

1 ng (nanogram) = 1×10^{-9} g, i.e. a billionth of a gram.

● What effect would increased GnRH secretion have on hormonal secretion by the anterior pituitary?

● GnRH stimulates secretion of luteinizing hormone (LH) and follicle-stimulating hormone (FSH) (Book 2, Section 3.5).

● What effects do FSH and LH have on hormone secretion in the testis? Refer to Book 2, Figure 3.10 if you need to refresh your memory.

● FSH and LH stimulate secretion of sex steroid hormones by the testis.

● What processes (other than gametogenesis) are initiated at puberty by testosterone?

● The surge of testosterone secretion at puberty stimulates growth in length and width of muscle fibres (Book 2, Section 4.8.5), leading to greater relative muscle mass in men than in women.

During and after puberty, Leydig cells respond to circulating LH by secreting sex steroids: large quantities of testosterone, about 4–10 mg per day, and small amounts of oestrogens. Some of the testosterone is converted into the more active steroid, *dihydrotestosterone* (*DHT*), by Sertoli cells, and this initiates and maintains spermatogenesis. Much of the testosterone is secreted into the bloodstream and some into the lymph. Circulating testosterone initiates masculinization during puberty, when physical features of adult males develop, including an enlarged larynx, body hair, beard, broad shoulders and relatively heavier skeletal and muscle mass. Throughout life male libido is maintained by circulating testosterone. Men who have no testosterone, e.g. because of removal of testes as treatment for testicular cancer, show a sharp decline in sexual thoughts, arousal and sexual activity. Treatment of such men with testosterone restores levels of sexual interest and activity. However, testosterone treatment has no such effect in men with normal levels of testosterone who have psychological problems that inhibit sexual activity. In a minority of infertile men, lack of testosterone is linked to lack of hypothalamic secretion of GnRH. Administration of subcutaneous pulses of GnRH to 11 such men, initiated spermatogenesis in 9 of them (Christiansen and Skakkebaek, 2002). Pulsatile administration and secretion of hormones prevents receptor downregulation (Book 2, Section 3.6.2), i.e. a loss of sensitivity of target cell receptors after continuous exposure to a signalling molecule.

Negative feedback plays a crucial role in the hormonal control of testosterone secretion, and spermatogenesis. Testosterone inhibits LH secretion, by direct action on the pituitary and indirectly, by reducing the frequency of GnRH pulses from the hypothalamus.

● Outline the molecular basis of hormone specificity, which is essentially the core mechanism for negative feedback. *Hint*: recall Book 2, Chapter 3.

● Although circulating hormones reach all body cells, only target cells with appropriate receptors can respond to particular hormones. Receptors, located in target cell membranes or inside cells, are globular protein molecules bearing specific binding sites for particular signalling molecules. Binding of a hormone to a receptor initiates the cell's response to the hormone.

Receptors in hypothalamic neurons initiate responses to specific hormones in the bloodstream, e.g. in response to elevated blood testosterone, receptors in the hypothalamus initiate reduction in GnRH secretion. The hormonal control of spermatogenesis is by means of negative feedback pathways, which can be represented by a flow chart (Figure 4.5).

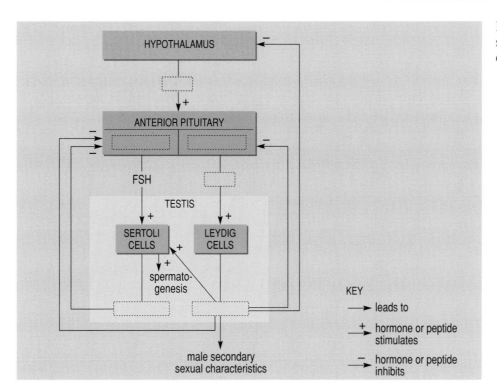

Figure 4.5   Flow chart summarizing the hormonal control of testicular function.

- Fill in the gaps as far as possible in Figure 4.5, a flow diagram that when complete, summarizes the hormonal control of testicular function. Leave gaps where you are unsure and fill them in as you read relevant parts of this section.

- The completed Figure 4.5 is provided overleaf (Figure 4.6), but we suggest that you delay viewing it until you have completed study of this section.

Your additions to Figure 4.5 show the three-tier hormonal control of spermatogenesis, and the crucial role of GnRH secreted by the hypothalamus. Receptors in target cells in the anterior pituitary respond to circulating GnRH by initiating secretion of FSH and LH. FSH is essential for spermatogenesis as it stimulates development of receptor proteins for testosterone in Sertoli cells (Section 4.2.1). In this way, testosterone inside the seminiferous tubules supports spermatogenesis. In turn, FSH secretion is inhibited by high levels of the cytokine inhibin, acting in an endocrine way, as it is secreted into the bloodstream by Sertoli cells. To some extent, FSH secretion is also inhibited by elevated blood testosterone.

- Now complete any remaining gaps in Figure 4.5; show the feedback exerted by inhibin and testosterone on hormone secretion by the anterior pituitary.

- See Figure 4.6 (overleaf).

Figure 4.6 Flow chart summarizing the hormonal control of testicular function. FSH is shown acting only on the Sertoli cells and LH is shown acting only on the Leydig cells. Testosterone is shown having both an endocrine and a paracrine role; it acts locally stimulating spermatogenesis and also acts hormonally, e.g by maintaining masculinization via effects on skin and skeleton.

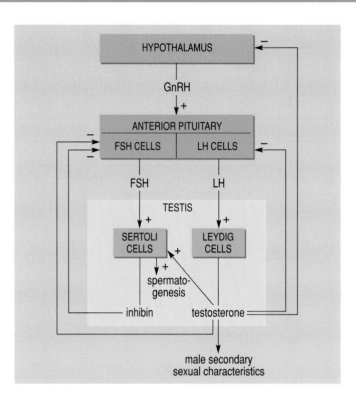

We have built up a detailed picture of the hormonal control of spermatogenesis. It is important to appreciate that, overall, the rates of secretion of GnRH, LH, FSH, testosterone and inhibin are quite constant from day to day in young men.

In contrast to the male reproductive system, that of the female produces just one, sometimes two and rarely three, mature gametes, oocytes, on a particular day, each month.

Consider the implications if synchronized spermatogenesis produced batches of mature sperm only once every 64 days. What would this pattern of sperm production mean for a couple wanting to have a baby (assuming a normal pattern of mature oocyte production in women)?

Whilst you ponder this question, consider the patterns of gametogenesis in another species. Eels are unusual fish, because when sexually mature both males and females migrate from their inland rivers to the sea. The males and females mature sexually during their long swim westwards to the Sargasso Sea in the Caribbean, where breeding takes place. Females spawn (i.e. lay their eggs), in synchrony and these eggs are fertilized by the group of males releasing sperm at the same time. This is the only time in their lives that these animals breed. Adult eels die after breeding and never return to their rivers. How has the eel's pattern of gametogenesis affected its breeding behaviour?

Red deer, living in northern temperate areas breed seasonally. Shortening day length in autumn stimulates secretion of GnRH by the hypothalamus, in turn switching on secretion of LH and FSH, and hence testosterone secretion in stags and oestrogen secretion in hinds. Mating occurs during October, the 'rutting' season for deer, and the hinds (female deer) are pregnant over winter. Each hind becomes fertile and willing to receive the stag's attention just once throughout the year. Although all hinds reach this point at a similar time of year the hinds in a group are not all fertile on the same day. Stags can mate with a succession of hinds and there is intense competition between males for access to the females. Consider how such a pattern of gamete maturation and breeding would affect human behaviour.

One reason for giving you this activity is to emphasize that there is much variation between species and that different physiological patterns of sperm production result in different behavioural patterns.

The implication of synchronized spermatogenesis every 64 days is that it would be difficult for a couple to conceive. Pulses of sperm production would occur only about six times per year. A woman produces a mature oocyte around the 15th day of the menstrual cycle, and that day would need to coincide with one of the few days in the year that viable sperm are available. One can speculate on how different our social and sexual lives would have been if the normal pattern of male gametogenesis produced mature sperm only six times a year. For example, mating is a waste of energy if there is *no* possibility of conception, so individuals who knew when they, and when potential partners were fertile would be favoured by natural selection.

We now move on to examine the sequence of cellular and tissue events involved in oocyte maturation, the menstrual cycle, and its tight control by the hypothalamic–pituitary axis.

Summary of Section 4.2

1   Location of the testes outside the body ensures that spermatogenesis takes place at an optimal temperature about 2–3°C cooler than body temperature.

2   Spermatogenesis takes place in the testes within coiled seminiferous tubules. Division of stem cells initiates spermatogenic cycles.

3   Groups of developing spermatozoa in seminiferous tubules are at different stages of development, so ensuring continuous production of spermatozoa.

4   The spermatogenic cycle takes 16 days. It takes a total of 64 days for a daughter cell of a stem cell to develop into a group of mature spermatozoa, so there are four successive waves of spermatogenesis in groups of developing spermatozoa derived from a stem cell.

5   The Sertoli cells provide nutrition and spatial organization for spermatogenesis. They also convert testosterone into the more active DHT (dihydrotestosterone).

6   Maturation of sperm takes place inside the epididymis, a collection of coiled tubes, where sperm are nourished by fructose and coated with glycoproteins.

7   Spermatogenesis requires endocrine support from FSH, and paracrine support from testosterone and dihydrotestosterone. Testosterone secretion by Leydig cells is controlled by LH via negative feedback pathways in the hypothalamic–pituitary axis. Target cell receptors mediate the negative feedback responses.

4.3 Oogenesis and the menstrual cycle

The female reproductive system (Figure 4.7) is more complex than that of males, as it includes the ovaries, whose role is to produce steroid hormones and gametes, and also the uterus, the site for implantation and development of the embryo. In this chapter our main focus is on the function of the paired ovaries. We examine how the pattern of release of steroid hormones controls growth, development and release of oocytes during the menstrual cycle.

Figure 4.7 The female reproductive system. The inset on the right-hand side shows both a complete view and a section of the fallopian tubes.

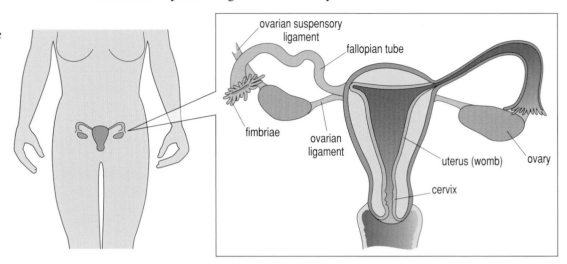

The ovaries are paired (Figure 4.7) and early in the development of a female embryo, there are oocyte stem cells inside each ovary. The stem cells divide by mitosis (Book 1, Section 2.9.3), forming millions of cells; before birth they all enter the first phase of meiosis. Those that survive become primary oocytes, which become enclosed by layers of cells from surrounding ovary tissue to form **primordial follicles** (Figure 4.8a). Meiosis then stops abruptly, leaving all oocytes in an arrested early stage of meiosis, when pairs of duplicated chromosomes are in intimate contact with each other (Figure 1.5). Large numbers of the arrested oocytes die, leaving about a million primordial follicles in the ovaries of a new-born baby girl, containing all of the oocytes in her ovaries that she will ever have. Unlike the testes, the ovaries remain in the abdominal cavity and are attached to the posterior abdominal wall.

Activation of secretion of GnRH by the hypothalamus initiates puberty around the age of 10–14, on average about 2 years earlier than in boys. Secretion of oestrogen by the ovaries regulates growth of female characteristics such as breasts and genitalia, and androgens control growth of female body hair. Menstrual cycles begin and initially may be irregular.

A menstrual cycle lasts about 28 days, although there is so much variation between women that cycles of 21–35 days are considered to be normal. A menstrual cycle can be split into two main phases, the **follicular phase** during which there is follicular development and growth, and following ovulation, the **luteal phase**. Ovulation, the release of a mature oocyte into a fallopian tube, takes place at around day 15. All stages of the menstrual cycle can only take place within a background of pulsatile release of GnRH from hypothalamic neurons into the bloodstream supplying the anterior pituitary (Book 2, Section 3.5).

GnRH stimulates secretion of FSH and LH from the anterior pituitary, which in turn stimulate the ovary to secrete sex steroids, including oestrogens and testosterone.

We now examine the menstrual cycle in more detail; inevitably the complex hormonal control of the cycle is an overarching theme throughout Sections 4.3.1 and 4.3.2.

4.3.1 The follicular phase

To understand the follicular phase, we need to go back to the second half (the luteal phase) of the previous menstrual cycle, when about 20 primordial follicles in each ovary start to grow slowly. The follicles lie within a glandular tissue, known as stroma (Figure 4.8a); endocrine cells there also secrete sex steroids. Each primordial follicle contains a primary oocyte surrounded by layers of follicular cells, which nourish and protect the developing oocyte. By the 5th–7th day of the following menstrual cycle, just one 'dominant' follicle (occasionally two or three) of the total of 40 growing follicles is 'selected' to grow further (Figure 4.8a), stimulated to grow by FSH. The mature follicle (c. 200–400 μm in diameter) is known as a Graafian follicle. The follicular cells secrete sex steroids – oestrogens (mainly oestradiol), progesterone and testosterone, most of which is then converted into oestradiol. These hormones are secreted into the bloodstream and also into follicular fluid where they have local paracrine actions. Oestrogens in follicular fluid stimulate follicular cells to proliferate.

Early in the menstrual cycle, a translucent layer of glycoproteins builds up, known as the **zona pellucida**, which separates the oocyte from the surrounding layers of follicular cells (Figure 4.8b).

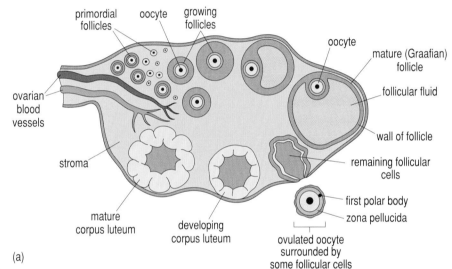

(a)

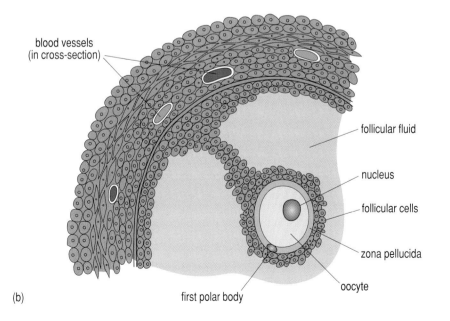

(b)

Figure 4.8   (a) Diagram of an ovary to show the development of a follicle and the production of a mature oocyte. Maturation proceeds clockwise from the top left. One of the primordial follicles is stimulated, and starts to grow. (b) Enlarged diagram showing the follicle containing the oocyte, much follicular fluid, and layers of follicular cells that nourish the oocyte. (a) shows that after ovulation, the remains of the follicle left inside the ovary develop into a structure called the corpus luteum, which secretes hormones that play a crucial role in maintaining the early stages of pregnancy (see text).

From an early stage in the menstrual cycle, follicular development depends on support from the anterior pituitary hormones, FSH and LH. Figure 4.9 shows the changes in levels of FSH, LH, oestradiol and progesterone during the menstrual cycle. Note how at the beginning of the cycle (days 1–6), when levels of circulating oestradiol (an oestrogen) are relatively low, the anterior pituitary responds by increasing release of FSH and LH.

● What kind of feedback is this? Why do low levels of oestradiol promote release of LH and FSH from the anterior pituitary?

● This is negative feedback in which FSH and LH release are inhibited by the negative feedback action of circulating oestrogen. When levels of circulating oestradiol are low, FSH and LH secretion increase, stimulating oestrogen secretion in the ovary.

FSH stimulates the growth and development of follicles. In early follicles, LH stimulates the cell layers to secrete oestrogens and to convert androgens, such as testosterone, into oestrogens. Follicular growth results in increased secretion of oestrogens.

Figure 4.10 is a flow chart that summarizes the endocrine control of the follicular phase of the menstrual cycle. The box for the ovary is enlarged so that details of hormonal action in the ovaries can be seen.

In Figure 4.10, inhibin secreted into the bloodstream by follicular cells is shown entering the bloodstream and inhibiting FSH secretion by the anterior pituitary. At the same time, oestrogens, in particular oestradiol, are released into the blood, and they exert feedback control of release of FSH and LH by the anterior pituitary. Oestrogens, especially oestradiol, also act paracrinally inside the ovary and bind to receptors in the follicular cells, which respond by proliferating, and secreting even more oestradiol (Figure 4.10).

● Is the paracrine action of oestrogens on granulosa cells an example of positive or negative feedback control of oestrogen secretion?

● It is positive feedback, because the action of oestrogen in promoting proliferation of follicular cells results in increased secretion of oestrogen.

The positive feedback pathway inside the ovary, whereby oestradiol stimulates further oestradiol output from follicular cells, results in ever-increasing blood levels of oestradiol (Figure 4.9b). Then around day 13 of the menstrual cycle, levels of oestradiol reach a threshold and trigger a *positive* feedback response to oestradiol in the anterior pituitary and hypothalmus, resulting in a surge of LH secretion by the anterior

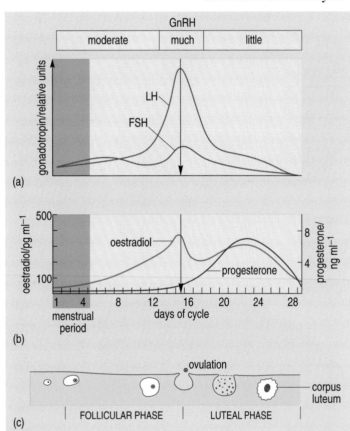

Figure 4.9   The pattern of blood levels of some hormones during the menstrual cycle in relation to GnRH levels and follicular development. The downward pointing arrow denotes the time of ovulation. The shaded area shows the timing of menstruation. (a) Levels of the gonadotropins LH and FSH during the menstrual cycle. (b) Levels of the steroid hormones oestradiol and progesterone during the menstrual cycle. (c) Stages of follicular development, ovulation and formation of the corpus luteum.

pituitary peaking at about day 15 of the cycle and coinciding with a smaller peak of FSH (Figure 4.9a). The surge in LH triggers terminal growth changes in the oocyte, which is expelled from the follicle at around day 15 of the menstrual cycle. The remains of the follicle left behind in the ovary develop into the **corpus luteum**, to which we return in Section 4.3.2.

We need to pause here and consider the events happening in the oocyte during the follicular phase. Every month just one (and occasionally two or three) oocyte resumes meiosis.

● At what stage of meiosis is development of the oocyte halted in the neonate?

● The oocyte is arrested at the first stage of meiosis.

Soon after the start of the surge of blood LH levels, the first division of meiosis resumes in the oocyte within the growing follicle. However, although half of the chromosomes go to each of the daughter cells, almost all of the cytoplasm is transferred to just one of the cells, the secondary oocyte. The other chromosomes are left in a small bag of cytoplasm, the first polar body (Figure 4.8b), which dies.

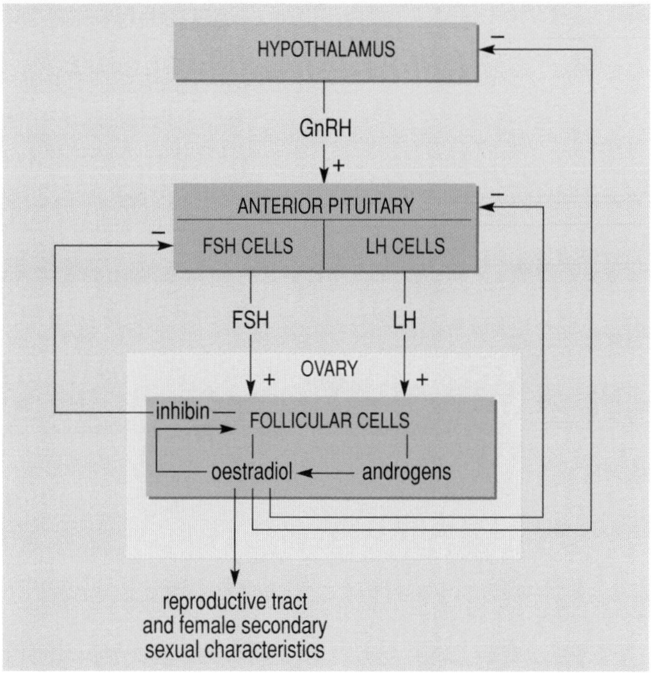

The oocyte is therefore a large cell, up to 120 μm in diameter; it continues meiosis with the chromosomes lining up at the equator, but the process is then arrested again. By now the follicle is bulging out from the surface of the ovary, and increased fluid pressure inside the follicle causes it to pop, and the oocyte enclosed by some follicular cells, is expelled from the ovary; this is ovulation. The frond-like **fimbriae** (Figure 4.7), sweeping over the surface of the ovary pick up the oocyte, which is transferred into a fallopian tube, where it is wafted gently downwards by the cilia on the epithelial cells that line it. Fertilization can take place in the fallopian tube if sperm are there.

Figure 4.10 A flow chart summarizing the hormonal control of the follicular phase of the menstrual cycle. Note the arrows in the follicular cells showing the conversion of androgens to oestradiol in these cells. Oestradiol exerts negative feedback on the anterior pituitary during the early follicular phase. (During the late follicular phase, when oestradiol levels are high, feedback becomes positive – not shown on this figure.)

4.3.2 The luteal phase

Following ovulation, follicle cells left in the ovary grow and develop into the corpus luteum and the menstrual cycle enters the luteal phase. The corpus luteum secretes large quantities of progesterone, and also inhibin, oestrogens and androgens. Progesterone and oestrogen maintain the lining of the uterus in an appropriate state for implantation of the early embryo. High blood progesterone depresses plasma FSH and LH by negative feedback, an effect enhanced by the endocrine action of inhibin.

● What is the consequence for ovarian function of low blood FSH levels during the luteal phase?

● Low levels of circulating FSH mean there is minimal stimulation of follicular growth. Therefore no new dominant follicle begins growth during the luteal phase.

Although levels of circulating oestradiol remain high after ovulation, at least up to day 24, (Figure 4.9b), an LH surge is not induced because the high levels of progesterone inhibit the positive feedback effect of high blood levels of oestradiol on the anterior pituitary. If there is no pregnancy, the corpus luteum breaks down, and oestrogen, progesterone and inhibin decline, removing the negative feedback effect on the pituitary. LH and FSH levels therefore rise, enabling initiation of growth of a dominant follicle or follicles and a new cycle.

We now return to the point in the menstrual cycle just after ovulation, and examine fertilization.

4.3.3 Fertilization

Within a minute of sexual intercourse, sperm can be detected in the cervix.

● Where do spermatozoa have to go in order to fertilize an oocyte?

● The spermatozoa need to swim through the cervix, up through the uterus, and into the fallopian tube (see Figure 4.7).

Relatively few spermatozoa manage to reach the cervix. They move through the uterus by wave-like beats of the tail, assisted by currents set up by uterine cilia. The sperm undergo **capacitation** in the uterus, a process taking several hours and involving removal of glycoproteins coating the surface of the sperm. Capacitation changes swimming movements to strong-whip-like beats of the tail that propel the sperm forwards. When sperm reach the entry point of the fallopian tubes, it is likely that they swim into the tube that contains the oocyte. Studies on the behaviour of sperm *in vitro*, suggest that follicular fluid contains chemicals that encourage sperm to swim towards the oocyte (Jaiswal et al., 1999).

The process of fertilization takes hours before it is completed. Initially, sperm cluster around an oocyte and attempt to penetrate the zona (Figure 4.11a, b). Capacitation initiates changes in the sperm head that facilitate penetration of the zona that encloses the oocyte. The first sperm cell that penetrates the oocyte fertilizes it, and no other sperm can penetrate the oocyte (Figures 4.11c–d). As a sperm cell penetrates the oocyte, it loses its tail (Figure 4.11d).

● What is the consequence of the loss of the sperm tail during fertilization? *Hint*: recall the events during the final stages of sperm development.

● Loss of the tail as the sperm penetrates the oocyte means that the mitochondria are left outside, which means that no paternal mitochondria are transmitted to the offspring.

Mitochondria contain their own DNA, which codes for mitochondrial structural proteins and proteins involved in glucose breakdown. As the fertilized oocyte, now a zygote, contains only maternal mitochondria, this means that all offspring inherit only maternal mitochondrial DNA. The second meiotic division of the oocyte is completed and one set of the maternal chromosomes is packaged into the second polar body, a small bag of cytoplasm, which is ejected from the much

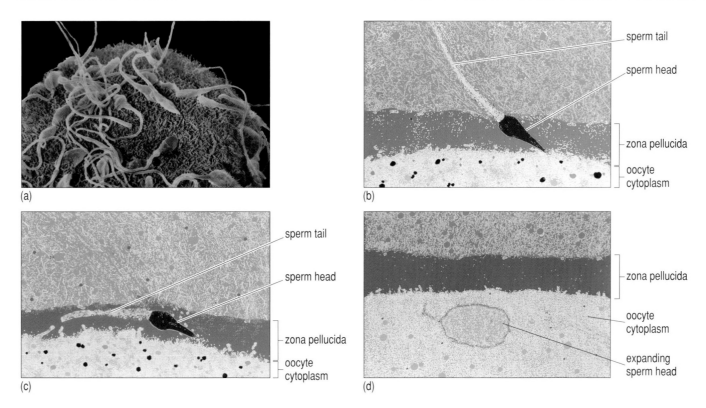

Figure 4.11 Sperm penetration into human oocytes *in vitro*. (a) A coloured scanning electron micrograph (SEM) of sperm on a human oocyte provides a three-dimensional view. The zona pellucida has a furry surface, coloured brown. Attached sperm (coloured yellow) attempt to penetrate the thick zona pellucida. Magnification: × 1600. (b) False colour transmission electron micrograph (TEM) of an oocyte during fertilization showing a single sperm that has just penetrated the zona pellucida, coloured aqua green, that encloses the oocyte. The sperm head, dark brown, is in the space between the zona and the oocyte. Orange blobs in the tail just below the sperm head are mitochondria. TEM enables viewing cells at extremely high magnification. (c) The sperm cell now sits in the space between the zona and the oocyte alongside the oocyte. This position depends on immunological recognition and attachment sites on the side of the sperm head. Once a sperm head has penetrated the oocyte, rapid thickening of the oocyte membrane prevents entry of competing sperm. (d) The sperm head inside the oocyte expands; the 23 chromosomes will begin to appear. The membranes of both sperm and oocyte nuclei (only the sperm nucleus is seen here), will break up releasing the chromosomes into the cytoplasm initiating the first mitosis. Magnification of (b)–(d): × 2000.

larger zygote. So the zygote now has two haploid nuclei, known as **pronuclei**, one from the oocyte and one from the sperm (Figure 4.12a, overleaf). Within the pronuclei, the haploid chromosomes synthesize DNA in preparation for mitosis (Book 1, Section 2.9.3). The pronuclear membranes break down, releasing two sets of chromosomes, one paternal and one maternal, so now the genetic material of the two parents has come together. The zygote then begins the first mitosis forming a two-celled embryo (Figure 4.12b).

4.3.4 The pre-implantation embryo

The human embryo remains in the fallopian tube for 3 days and undergoes mitosis there. During this time the embryo does not grow in size, so that with each successive cell division, the size of the cells, known as **blastomeres**, decreases (Figure 4.12c–e).

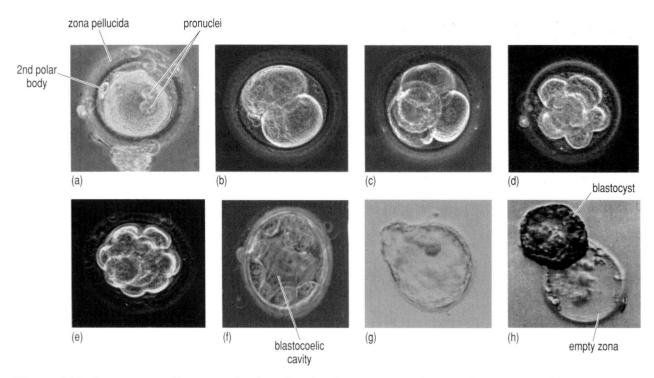

Figure 4.12 Some stages of human preimplantation development. At each stage, the zona pellucida can be seen. (a) A fertilized oocyte inside the zona. There are two pronuclei inside the oocyte and two polar bodies below the zona. (b) The two-cell stage. (c) The four-cell stage. (d) The eight-cell stage. (e)The 16-cell stage in which the blastomeres are flattened and compacted. (f) Early blastocyst stage, in which a blastocoelic cavity forms. (g) Blastocyst hatching through the zona pellucida. (h) Blastocyst hatched, with empty zona lying beneath it and partly covered by it.

Essentially the cell division is cleavage, in which the cytoplasm is divided between daughter cells, with no increase in the total amount of cytoplasm (see Book 1 Section 1.6). These cell divisions restore the normal cell nucleus : cytoplasm ratio. At 3.5 days after fertilization, the embryo enters the uterus, where cell divison continues so that at 4.5 days it has reached the 32–64 cell stage, a blastocyst, in which the cells form a ball enclosing a cavity (Figure 4.12f).

In rare cases, the embryo remains in the fallopian tube, and develops into a blastocyst which implants in the wall of the fallopian tube. This is known as an **ectopic pregnancy** and is dangerous for the mother, as the wall of the fallopian tube will rupture as the embryo grows. Rare cases of ectopic pregnancy involve embryos attached in the abdominal cavity. The incidence of ectopic pregnancy is about 1 in 50 pregnancies but is increasing due to an increased incidence of damaged fallopian tubes. This damage is largely a result of infection from sexually transmitted diseases.

Case Report 4.1 Ectopic pregnancy

Penny, a 21-year-old call centre worker, arrived in A&E one Thursday afternoon. She was 12 weeks pregnant but had become increasingly aware of lower abdominal pain. In fact she felt so unwell that morning that her friend Karen agreed to accompany her to see her local GP. After examining Penny the GP requested her to go straight to A&E, ascertaining that her friend could take her on the very short drive. He told Penny that tests were needed quickly to confirm why she was feeling the pain.

On arrival, Penny had baseline observations of temperature, pulse, respirations (breathing rate) and blood pressure recorded and these were all within normal parameters, though the nurse recorded that Penny looked rather pale and was in some discomfort. A pregnancy test was taken and the results confirmed the pregnancy. Penny was then seen by an obstetrician who ordered an ultrasound scan, but this showed lack of uterine pregnancy. The obstetrician decided to admit Penny to the gynaecological ward.

Penny was admitted to a four-bedded ward. The obstetrician explained that the tests indicated ectopic pregnancy and that in this condition the pregnancy develops not in the uterus but (usually) in the fallopian tube. Penny asked if this would mean she would lose the baby and was told this would be so. However, it was explained that because the fallopian tube may rupture, internal bleeding could reduce circulating blood volume so much that it causes shock (known as hypovolaemic shock; Book 3, Section 2.6.5). Ectopic pregnancies cannot continue to term (birth) so removal of the developing embryo and placenta are necessary to save the life of the mother. Penny signed a consent form for this surgery. Her friend Karen, who had been present throughout, rang Penny's partner who arranged to come to the ward. The staff nurse on the ward monitored Penny carefully, taking her respirations, pulse, blood pressure and temperature at regular intervals, observing for the early signs of hypovolaemic shock. She also closely observed Penny's general condition, particularly looking for increased levels of pain, feelings of being faint, or fainting, and referred pain to the shoulder (Book 2, Section 2.1.2). All these symptoms are indications of rupturing of the fallopian tube. The staff nurse ensured that Penny and her partner understood what the obstetrician had said, and gently supported them. Penny was now becoming upset at the thought of losing the pregnancy.

Penny was prepared for surgery in the usual way; she had an intravenous cannula inserted into the back of her hand and was advised to take no fluids or food since she was scheduled for surgery later that evening. **Laparoscopy** was performed, in which a thin lighted tube with a tiny camera is inserted into a small cut in the abdomen and tiny instruments at the end of the tube are used to remove the fallopian tube and the embryo. Postoperatively, Penny recovered from the surgery very quickly. The observations taken during monitoring remained within her normal range. Within 24 hours she was ready to return home. Penny remained upset but felt a little better because the staff acknowledged that ectopic pregnancy is a difficult experience. As well as recovering from the operation, Penny had to cope with the loss of her pregnancy and the loss of part of her fertility. Penny asked if she would be able to conceive and have a normal pregnancy in the future. She was told the chances of a repeat ectopic are about 10%, so 9 out of 10 future pregnancies would be in the womb. Penny was given an advice and information booklet before discharge and her continuing care passed to the primary health care team.

From fertilization to blastocyst stage, the embryo remains enclosed in the zona pellucida (Figure 4.12a–f). The zona is a protective capsule that prevents the blastomeres from separating during early cleavage. However, if the embryo does split into two during early cleavage, monozygotic twins develop from two genetically identical embryos. If the embryo splits from 4–8 days after conception, each twin has its own **amniotic sac**, a sac of fluid enclosed by protective membranes, but the twins share one placenta. About 30% of monozygotic twins each have their own placenta.

The blastocyst obtains its nutrition and oxygen from uterine secretions. Before implantation at 7–9 days, the blastocyst must 'hatch' out of the zona pellucida (Figure 4.12g–h).

When the blastocyst is in the uterus, it signals its presence by secreting a hormone known as **human chorionic gonadotropin (hCG)**, which has similar effects to those of LH, in that it maintains the corpus luteum.

● Why is it important to have a functional corpus luteum during early pregnancy?

○ The corpus luteum secretes oestrogen and large amounts of progesterone, which inhibit secretion of FSH and LH by the pituitary. If the corpus luteum were to die, steroid hormone levels would plummet, and FSH secretion would increase, initiating growth of a new dominant follicle and a new menstrual cycle and the loss of the early embryo.

Raised hCG levels in the blood and urine 18–30 days after the last menstrual period are used to detect pregnancy at a very early stage.

Implantation of the embryo involves invasion of the uterine lining by the placenta and is followed by rapid development of an amniotic sac around the embryo.

● Occasionally, embryos may split into two at between 8 and 12 days. Suggest the consequences in terms of the embryo itself, the placenta and the amniotic sac.

○ Monozygotic twins will develop and they will share not only a placenta but also develop inside the same amniotic sac, because by 8 days after conception, implantation has occurred and one amniotic sac has developed.

In the UK about 1 in 35 babies born are twins or triplets (Multiple Births Foundation, 2004); of these most are twins. One-third of twins are monozygotic, and two-thirds are dizygotic, formed by the fertilization of two separate oocytes by two independent sperm.

We can leave implantation and development of the embryo at this stage, as we have sufficient information to move on to examine how understanding of the ovarian cycle and fertilization enabled development of contraceptive pills. We also examine the problems that cause infertility and how they may be resolved by the use of *in vitro* fertilization (IVF), for production of a healthy embryo with the potential to develop into a healthy baby.

Summary of Section 4.3

1   The female reproductive system has three major functions: production of haploid oocytes; secretion of sex steroid hormones; and provision of a uterine lining suitable for implantation and development of an embryo.

2   The ovaries of a new-born baby girl contain all the oocytes she will ever have, about a million, in an arrested early stage of meiosis inside primordial follicles.

3   Menstrual cycles begin at puberty and each lasts for about 28 days, controlled by complex hormonal interactions within the hypothalamic–pituitary axis and the ovaries.

4   The follicular phase of a menstrual cycle begins with growth of one or two dominant follicles, stimulated by FSH. About half way through the cycle, a positive feedback response of the pituitary to high oestrogen levels releases a surge of LH that triggers resumption of meiosis in the oocyte, expulsion of the first polar body, and ovulation.

5   The luteal phase begins as remaining follicle cells in the ovary develop into the corpus luteum, which secretes progesterone and oestrogen; these steroids suppress secretion of FSH and LH by the pituitary.

6   The oocyte is wafted through one of the fallopian tubes, where fertilization may take place. Fertilization takes several hours, beginning after sperm penetration of the oocyte.

7   After the two sets of chromosomes, maternal and paternal, come together, the first mitosis occurs forming the two-celled embryo. Further mitoses in the early embryo lead to development of the blastocyst, which has to 'hatch' out of the zona before it can be implanted into the mother's uterine lining.

4.4 Contraception: controlled suppression of gametogenesis

Contraception, or prevention of pregnancy, helps to promote the birth and growth of healthy babies by enabling prospective parents to plan for pregnancy when they have sufficient resources for providing for both healthy pregnancy and good baby care. The spacing of pregnancies at intervals long enough to allow the mother to recover from pregnancy, childbirth and breastfeeding promotes the health of both babies and mother.

Understanding the endocrine control of the menstrual cycle facilitated the development of contraception by means of suitable steroids, in particular, by oestrogen and **progestins**, which are progesterone analogues. The original research dates from the late 1940s, when Carl Djerassi and a few colleagues formed Syntex, a chemical firm, based in Mexico. The researchers were interested in developing steroid chemistry, and a major breakthrough for them was Djerassi's discovery that the inedible Mexican wild yam is a rich source of compounds with a sterol nucleus (Book 2, Box 3.1). One of the steroids extracted from that yam, diosgenin, provided the raw material for synthesis of norethindrone, an orally active progestin. This formed the basis of the first birth control pills. After being tested in animals the compound was tested in clinical trials in women in Puerto Rico, USA and Haiti. The success of the trials led to the marketing of Enovid, a pill containing norethindrone, combined with a small amount of synthetic oestrogen.

● What would be the effect of persistent high levels of norethindrone, a progestin, in the bloodstream?

● Progesterone and its analogues suppress ovulation by negative feedback action on FSH and LH secretion by the anterior pituitary. The positive feedback effect of oestrogen on the pituitary is also suppressed (Section 4.3.2).

Initially, in 1957, Enovid was used not as a contraceptive, but as treatment for disorders of menstruation. For example, Enovid was used to treat endometriosis, in which pieces of uterine lining become attached to internal organs such as the intestine and ovary, where they continue responding to the menstrual cycle, causing pain and in the long term scarring and possible blockage of fallopian tubes. Amenorrhea, lack of menstrual cycles, and menorrhagia, heavy bleeding during menstruation, were also treated by Enovid. Later the steroids were approved for use as oral contraceptives after the reassuring outcomes of surveys comparing the risks of taking the pill with risks involved in pregnancy and childbirth. Critics pointed out that if Enovid use had been compared with the risks of using condoms and diaphragms, its safety would not have looked so good. Nevertheless, by the end of 1964 more than 4 million women in the UK had used the steroid pills, which came to be known as 'the pill'. The first versions of the pill contained oestrogen as well as progestins, and similar versions are in use today, known as combined oral contraceptives (COCs). In some women side-effects of the pill include those associated with early pregnancy, such as headache, swollen tender breasts, weight gain and lethargy.

The oestrogen in COCs promotes additional negative feedback on the pituitary and development of progesterone receptors, which make the progesterone in the pill even more effective. These pills are taken from day 1 to day 21 of a cycle.

● Suggest the effect of taking COC pills for 21 days on the pituitary and ovary.

● The output of gonadotropins LH and FSH, follicular growth and ovarian oestrogen are completely suppressed.

From days 22–28 the pill is not taken and the endometrium (uterine lining) breaks down, resulting in withdrawal bleeding that resembles menstruation.

● What is the effect on the pituitary and ovary of withdrawal of steroids for 7 days?

● The hypothalamus and pituitary are stimulated, resulting in rising secretion of FSH and LH and hence follicular development.

Failure to resume taking the pill after 7 days off can result in pregnancy, as ovulation is imminent. This can be deduced from Figure 4.13.

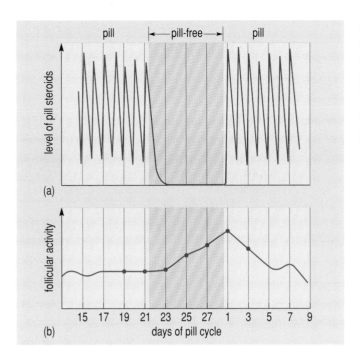

Figure 4.13 Blood steroid levels and follicular activity during use of the combined oral contraceptive. Pill-taking days and pill-free days are marked. The green-shaded area indicates withdrawal bleeding. (a) The peaks of blood steroid levels demonstrate the episodic nature of steroid intake. Note how steroid levels plummet when pill-taking ceases. (b) Follicular activity measured by ultrasound scan, effectively a measure of follicular size.

● Describe the effect indicated in Figure 4.13 of the break in pill-taking on blood steroid levels and follicular activity.

● Pill steroid levels plummet as soon as pill-taking ceases and follicular activity resumes quickly, with follicular size peaking at the end of day 28.

This treatment programme (regimen) is described as monocyclic. For some women who find it difficult to cope with a monthly bleed, a bicyclic regimen may be recommended; this involves 42 days of pill-taking followed by a 7-day break.

The regimen selected is that best suited to the individual needs of a woman with the fewest side-effects. There are many brands of pill available now, each containing different levels and balances of progestin and oestrogen, and a suitable one can usually (but not always), be found for each individual woman. Progestin-only pills, known as POPs, are taken daily without breaks or are administered by means of a subcutaneous (under the skin) depot that is replenished by injection. Progestins work by reducing sugar and protein levels in cervical fluid, thus reducing sperm viability. Progestin-induced thickening of cervical mucus and suppression of cilia in the fallopian tubes make it difficult for sperm to penetrate. In about 20% of users, ovulation is suppressed. Side-effects are few but irregular bleeding may occur, which may be unacceptable for some women.

Life-threatening effects of oral contraceptives were identified as long ago as 1967. Increased risks of certain cancers have been associated with taking steroid contraceptive pills. For example, a slight increase in the risk of breast cancer has been reported in women who have taken the pill for several years before the age of 25. The risk of deep vein thrombosis (DVT), for non pill-taking women is about 5 in 100 000. For those women taking the pill, the risk is increased by 2–6 fold (Gomes and Deitcher, 2004), up to 10–30 in 100 000. However, pregnancy carries the highest risk of DVT, about 70 in 100 000.

● Compare the risk of DVT in unplanned pregnancy with that of taking the pill.

◐ If the use of unreliable contraceptive methods resulted in unplanned pregnancy, a woman would be at a 2–7 times higher risk of thrombosis during her pregnancy than if she were not pregnant and taking the pill.

For older women, a history of cardiovascular disease or blood clots are contraindications for use of the pill. However, a recent extensive study involving 160 000 women (Victory et al., 2004) suggests that in women using the pill for at least a year, the risk of cardiovascular disease of any kind is reduced by 10%. There is no doubt that pill taking is beneficial for most women in reducing the risk of pregnancy and enabling family planning. However, the risk of thrombosis when taking the pill is increased by smoking and obesity, so women can reduce the risks of pill taking by not smoking and by avoiding obesity.

There have been attempts to suppress spermatogenesis by manipulation of the hypothalamic–pituitary axis, but so far there has been little success. Suppression of GnRH and gonadotropin release via negative feedback depresses testosterone secretion, reducing libido and expression of masculinization (Section 4.2.2). Administration of a long-lasting synthetic testosterone, known as the 'male pill' does reduce sperm count to very low levels, of around 3×10^6 sperm ml^{-1} semen, compared with the fertile range of $50–150 \times 10^6$ sperm ml^{-1} semen.

● Suggest a mechanism for the action of the 'male pill' on sperm production.

◐ High blood testosterone levels inhibit secretion of FSH and LH. Testosterone is essential for spermatogenesis, but without FSH there is no development of receptors for testosterone in the testis and hence no stimulus for spermatogenesis.

Side-effects of the early version of the male pill included acne, oily skin and weight gain, which are sufficiently unpleasant to persuade men to stop taking the pills. Newer versions of the male pill containing a progestin have been produced and are being tested, but they require supplementation with testosterone.

In this section, we have seen how gametogenesis can be suppressed by appropriate hormonal treatment for the purpose of contraception. In the following section we examine how the menstrual cycle can be manipulated by use of hormonal treatments to correct infertility in women.

Summary of Section 4.4

1 Understanding the hormonal control of the menstrual cycle led to the development of contraceptive pills based on synthetic progestins and oestrogens. The first progestin to be synthesized was derived from an inedible yam, and named 'norethindrone'.

2 Progestins such as progesterone suppress ovulation by negative feedback action and anti-positive feedback action on the pituitary and hypothalamus, even if oestrogen levels are high.

3 Progesterone and progestins thicken cervical mucus, and reduce the number of cilia in the fallopian tubes, thereby suppressing sperm penetration. Sugar and protein levels in uterine and fallopian tube fluids decline in response to progestins, which generally create an unfavourable environment for sperm.

4   Currently there are many versions of the pill and most women can find one that is suitable, with few side-effects. Combined oral contraceptives, COCs, contain progestin and oestrogen. POPs are progestin-only pills.

5   All versions of the pill have to be taken in accordance with a strict timetable; missing just one day can result in ovulation and high risk of pregnancy.

6   So far, a usable male 'pill' has not been found, but pills based on progestin with injections of testosterone are being tested.

4.5 Infertility and its treatment in women

In Section 4.1 we learned that about 10–15% of couples fail to conceive within 1–2 years of trying, a situation defined as clinical subfertility. In women, problems with either or both of gametogenesis and fertilization can reduce or abolish the chances of pregnancy. Ovulation failure due either to absent or infrequent menstrual cycles accounts for 20% of reported cases of difficulty in conception. Other problems that prevent conception in women include blockage of fallopian tubes and polycystic ovarian syndrome (Section 4.5.2).

● Why does blockage of the fallopian tubes prevent conception?

◐ At ovulation the mature oocyte is expelled from the ovary, swept up by the finger-like fimbriae and transferred into one of the fallopian tubes. After intercourse, spermatozoa swim to the fallopian tubes where fertilization takes place. If the fallopian tube is blocked, spermatozoa cannot reach the oocyte, and the oocyte can never reach the uterus.

The remaining cases of infertility are grouped as 'unexplained infertility' as no cause can be found. We can now examine some of the causes of infertility in women in more detail, and explore some of the available treatment options.

4.5.1 Blockage of fallopian tubes

Damaged fallopian tubes may be blocked or blocked and swollen with fluid. Both conditions can be detected by laparoscopy (Case Report 4.1). For detecting tubular blockages, a dye, methylene blue, is infused into the uterus via the cervix and the location and movement of the dye can be monitored. X-ray diagnosis may also be used, and in this procedure, known as *hysterosalpingography*, the radiographer infuses a radio-opaque dye into the uterus (Figure 4.14) to produce a hysterosalpingogram.

● How can a radiographer diagnose tubular blockage from a hysterosalpingogram (Figure 4.14b)?

◐ If the tubes were open as normal, the radio-opaque dye would flow into the tubes and out via the fimbriae, and spread into the abdominal cavity (Figure 4.14a). If the tubes were blocked the radio-opaque dye would either travel part-way up the tubes or remain in the uterus, depending on the location of the blockage (Figure 4.14b).

Tubular blockage or damage usually results from a sexually transmitted pelvic infection such as gonorrhea or chlamydia, that causes **pelvic inflammatory**

Figure 4.14
(a) Hysterosalpingogram from a woman with open fallopian tubes. The radio-opaque medium is leaking out of the fallopian tubes into the abdominal cavity.
(b) Hysterosalpingogram from a woman with blocked fallopian tubes – note the radio-opaque medium trapped inside a swollen blocked tube.

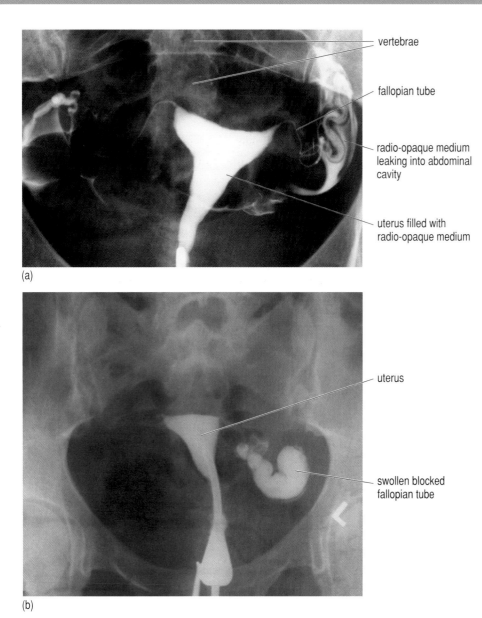

(a)

vertebrae

fallopian tube

radio-opaque medium leaking into abdominal cavity

uterus filled with radio-opaque medium

uterus

swollen blocked fallopian tube

(b)

disease **(PID)**, in which the uterus, fallopian tubes and ovaries can be affected. PID damages the cilia lining the fallopian tubes and blocks transport of both oocytes and sperm. Termination of pregnancy is followed by PID in about 10% of cases. Currently the prevalence of PID is estimated at about 2% in women of reproductive age seen by GPs per year (Practical Support for Clinical Governance PRODIGY, 2004). The exact incidence is unknown as many women with PID are asymptomatic and are therefore unaware that they have the condition. A study of 1309 women with PID showed that 10% of these women had tubular blockage, compared with none in the control group. PID infections can also cause permanent scarring and adhesions that restrict movement of the fallopian tube, or block the ends of the tubes. Surgery to repair and free the tubes is attempted initially in most patients, and has success rates of about 30–40%, but these are lower for those with severe tubular damage. For patients with severe tubular damage, currently the best treatment option is *in vitro* fertilization (IVF), in which oocytes are harvested from the ovaries and fertilized by spermatozoa in a dish containing a sterile nutrient solution.

Normally only one or rarely two, oocytes are released from the ovaries each month. For the purpose of IVF, practitioners like to have at least five and preferably up to ten oocytes available for harvesting.

● Examine Figure 4.9 and suggest an explanation for the development and release of only one oocyte and rarely two during each menstrual cycle.

● FSH stimulates follicular development, but at around day 9 of the cycle, FSH levels begin to drop so it is likely that the relatively low levels of FSH can support continued growth and development of just one, sometimes two, follicles.

In order to increase the number of developing follicles, the patient's own menstrual cycle is shut down and hormonal treatments are used to impose a controlled cycle that results in maturation of up to 10 follicles. A cycle of treatment takes about 5 weeks and begins on day 21 of the woman's menstrual cycle. On that day the patient is treated with a GnRH agonist such as *nafarelin,* administered by nasal spray, or *buserelin*, administered by injection.

● What effect would a GnRH agonist have on target tissues for GnRH?

● An agonist is a molecule that mimics the action of a signalling molecule. So a GnRH agonist will have the same action as GnRH on target cells. The GnRH agonist will stimulate the anterior pituitary to secret FSH and LH.

GnRH agonists have long half-lives (Book 2, Section 3.9), so within a few days the GnRH agonist *prevents* the woman from secreting her own FSH and LH secretion and, therefore, oestradiol secretion is also suppressed.

● Why does the persistent presence of a GnRH agonist shut down secretion of FSH and LH from the anterior pituitary?

● Receptors for GnRH in the anterior pituitary cells lose their sensitivity to GnRH unless its pattern of secretion is pulsatile. This is receptor downregulation (Section 4.2, and Book 2, Section 3.6) and in the anterior pituitary, this blunts the response of pituitary endocrine cells, which shut down secretion of LH and FSH.

An example of a calendar for a controlled cycle is provided in Figure 4.15 (overleaf). Details of treatments are tailored for individual women but the principles are the same in all cases. Synarel (a GnRH agonist) is taken as two nasal sprays per day for 17 days. Self-administration of FSH is by means of daily subcutaneous injections using an auto-injector.

● When did FSH injections begin for this woman?

● FSH injections begin on the 9th day of Synarel treatment.

● What effect on the ovary would you predict for the daily FSH injections?

● FSH stimulates follicular growth and secretion of steroid hormones by the ovary. Continuing high levels of FSH would promote growth and development of follicles.

From day 6 of FSH treatment a daily ultrasound scan is used to monitor follicle number and size (Figure 4.15).

FEBRUARY 2003

SUNDAY	MONDAY	TUESDAY	WEDNESDAY	THURSDAY	FRIDAY	SATURDAY
				Collect Synarel prescription		**1** _Day 19 of menstrual cycle_
2 _Day 20 of menstrual cycle_	**3** _Day 21_ Started on Synarel nose spray; 09:00 & 22:00	**4** _Day 22_ Synarel 09:00 & 22:00	**5** _Day 23_ Synarel 09:00 & 22:00	**6** _Day 24_ Synarel 09:00 & 22:00 Bad headache; no sleep	**7** _Day 25_ Synarel 09:00 & 22:00 Headache; day off work	**8** _Day 26_ Synarel 09:00 & 22:00
9 _Day 27_ Synarel 09:00 & 22:00	**10** _Day 1 (menstrual period starts)_ Synarel 09:00 & 22:00	**11** Synarel 09:00 & 22:00 11:00 clinic scan & blood test & another lesson in injecting myself My 1st — yuk FSH injection!	**12** Synarel 09:00 & 22:00 09:30 FSH injection	**13** Synarel 09:00 & 22:00 09:30 FSH injection	**14** Synarel 09:00 & 22:00 09:30 FSH injection Headache	**15** Synarel 09:00 & 22:00 09:30 FSH injection Headache and feel bloated
16 Synarel 09:00 & 21:00 09:30 FSH injection 11:00 clinic for scan & blood test bloating is vile	**17** Synarel 09:00 & 21:00 09:30 FSH injection 11:00 clinic for scan & blood test bloating bad today	**18** Synarel 09:00 & 21:00 09:30 FSH injection 11:00 clinic for scan & blood test always bloated	**19** Synarel 09:00 & 21:00 09:30 FSH injection 11:00 clinic for scan & blood test 22:00 hCG injection	**20** Feeling very restless and bloated Couldn't sleep	**21** DON'T EAT 09:30 clinic for egg retrieval; survived the sedation. Sperm collection for IVF	**22** Progesterone pessary. Clinic checking eggs for fertilization feeling very sore and can't stand up straight but very happy!
23 Progesterone pessary. Better today — have 6 good embryos	**24** 10:00 Clinic for 2 embryo transfer 18:00 progesterone pessary	**25** Progesterone pessary	**26** Progesterone pessary	**27** Progesterone pessary	**28** Progesterone pessary	

MARCH 2003

SUNDAY	MONDAY	TUESDAY	WEDNESDAY	THURSDAY	FRIDAY	SATURDAY
						1 *Progesterone pessary*
2 *Progesterone pessary*	**3** *Progesterone pessary*	**4** *Progesterone pessary*	**5** *Progesterone pessary*	**6** *Progesterone pessary*	**7** *Pregnancy test today!*	

Figure 4.15 Nathalie's* calendar, showing timings for stages of her IVF treatment. Each IVF clinic has their own procedures, modified for individual women. Treatment calendars will not be the same for every clinic and/or every woman.

- Why are regular scans (ultrasound monitoring) of the stimulated ovaries essential?

- Regular scans check the growth of follicles (and therefore oocytes) so that ovulation does not take place before the oocytes are harvested.

When the follicles have reached an optimum size, an injection of hCG (human chorionic gonadotropin) is given, which mimics the effect of LH on the developing follicles and stimulates maturation of the oocytes.

The oocytes are harvested about 36 hours after the hCG injection, when they are almost ready for ovulation. A needle attached to a vaginal ultrasound probe is inserted into the vagina. The needle is used to probe the surface of the ovary and suck out oocytes from large follicles that bulge out from the ovary surface. The process is monitored continuously by vaginal ultrasound scanning. The patient is sedated during this procedure. The harvested oocytes are washed into a dish containing warm culture medium. Progesterone is then administered to the woman by means of pessaries or by vaginal cream.

* Not the woman's real name.

● Suggest the purpose of progesterone treatment at this stage.

● Progesterone is essential for successful implantation and maintenance of the pregnancy. Removal of the oocytes mimics ovulation and normally after ovulation the corpus luteum develops and starts to secrete progesterone.

On the morning of oocyte collection, the male partner is asked to produce a sperm sample by masturbation.

● Why are freshly ejaculated sperm not capable of fertilizing an oocyte?

● Sperm are incapable of fertilization until they have been capacitated. Enzymes in uterine secretions remove the glycoproteins that coat ejaculated sperm, which initiates active swimming movements and cause changes in the sperm head that enable penetration of the zona (Section 4.3.3).

Washing sperm in suitable media *in vitro* fulfils the same function as uterine capacitation. About 5–6 hours after oocyte collection, sperm are mixed with the oocytes in the dish, and the following day the oocytes are checked for signs of fertilization. If fertilization has occurred the embryos are transferred to the woman's uterus 48 hours after oocyte collection, by which time the embryos consist of four or eight cells. At the time of writing (2005), new guidelines published by the Human Fertilization and Embryology Authority (HFEA, 2004) have restricted the number of transferred embryos to two, in order to reduce the risk of multiple pregnancies in women less than 40 years old.

4.5.2 Disorders of ovulation

Disorders of ovulation include *amenorrhea*, lack of menstrual cycles, and *oligomenorrhea*, infrequent cycles. The underlying causes require investigation and may respond to medication. Two types of medication are used. Clomiphene citrate (usually known as clomiphene) is an anti-oestrogenic drug that stimulates the anterior pituitary to release FSH. It is prescribed in pill form to be taken on days 1–5 of the woman's menstrual cycle. If the woman does not have regular menstrual cycles, they may be induced first by treatment with birth control pills prior to clomiphene treatment. Initially, low doses of clomiphene are prescribed; if this does not induce ovulation the dose is increased. If ultrasound scans indicate good follicle development, the couple are advised to have intercourse or to opt for intrauterine insemination.

Ovulation is induced in about 50–80% of women treated with clomiphene but only about 40% of these women become pregnant. It is possible that oocytes produced in response to clomiphene treatment are of poorer quality than those produced in normal cycles. Clomiphene also changes the quality and quantity of cervical mucus, which may reduce the chances of fertilization. One problem with clomiphene treatment is that there is a risk of multiple pregnancies, in which three or more embryos develop.

If clomiphene treatment does not work, injections of FSH are given. The injections begin early in the menstrual cycle and continue for 8–14 days until one or more mature follicles can be detected by ultrasound. An injection of hCG follows, which induces ovulation about 36 hours later. About 90% of the women treated with FSH ovulate, and 15% of patients treated per month become pregnant when this treatment is combined with intrauterine insemination. Unfortunately, ovarian hyperstimulation, which causes abdominal pain, enlarged ovaries and abdominal oedema, can occur with these treatments. Multiple pregnancies are also a risk, and pregnancies of three or more fetuses occur in 4% of women.

Polycystic ovarian syndrome

Polycystic ovarian syndrome (PCOS) is the most common cause of ovulation failure in women. The ovaries typically contain numerous small immature follicles. Laparoscopy of polycystic ovaries reveals that they are enlarged and contain multiple cysts, about 2–9 mm in diameter, causing their polycystic appearance (Figure 4.16b).

● Suggest what could be the cause of the lack of ovulation in the woman who has PCOS.

● Ovulation only occurs when the follicle and the oocyte within it are mature. Small follicles suggest immature follicles which cannot undergo ovulation.

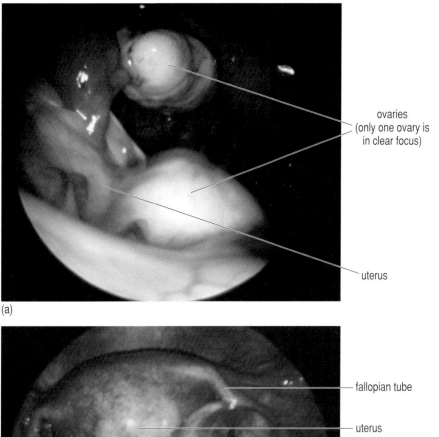

(a)

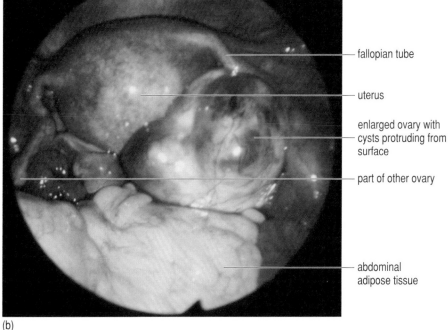

(b)

Figure 4.16   (a) Image of a normal ovary as seen during laparoscopy. (b) Image of a typical polycystic ovary as seen during laparoscopy.

● Examine Figure 4.16b and describe the ovary from a woman who has PCOS. Examine Figure 4.16a, also a laparoscopic view, for comparison, and describe the ovaries of the woman who was ovulating normally.

● The ovary from the woman with PCOS contains cysts bulging from the white surface and is enlarged. In contrast the ovaries in Figure 4.16a, from a woman who ovulates normally, are smooth and white.

Case Report 4.2 Polycystic ovarian syndrome (PCOS)

Norma is 23 and works in a solicitor's office. She has been married to Brian for 3 years and they have been trying for a baby for 2 years. Norma knew that she was overweight, in fact obese. Her weight had been within normal parameters until she was about 15 when she began to put on a significant amount of weight. By the time she was 20 she weighed 95 kg and at 5 ft 5 ins (1.65 m) had a BMI of 35 and was therefore considered obese. During her late teens Norma began to develop acne on her trunk and neck. She also began to develop excess hair on her face, neck and trunk but was losing hair on her head. Norma became quiet, anxious and described herself as depressed.

At the behest of Brian, Norma went to see her GP who eventually confirmed that Norma had polycystic ovarian syndrome. He explained that there is often no simple proof that a woman has the syndrome and it has been estimated that 25% of females have polycystic ovaries, with about 80% having one or more of the symptoms of the syndrome. In addition about 80% of women with normal ovaries can also experience one or more of the symptoms. Diagnosis of the syndrome is primarily made on a woman's medical history and presence of several classical signs. Patients with PCOS are often overweight (the weight being centred around the midsection of the body), have irregular or no menstrual cycles, excess hair on face and body (with thinning on top of the head), and adult acne. Blood tests to measure hormone levels can aid diagnosis, and when the disease is present it can involve elevated insulin levels, insulin resistance or diabetes. Previously known as Stein–Leventhal syndrome, polycystic ovarian syndrome is a disorder that includes numerous benign cysts forming on the ovaries under a thick white covering (Figure 4.16b). It is more common in women under 30 years old and is due to an abnormal production of LH and FSH. Imbalance of these hormones prevents the ovaries from releasing an egg each month. It also results in an abnormally high production of the male hormone testosterone by the ovaries.

Norma was encouraged to lose weight and referred to the local hospital for advice and possible treatment to help her become pregnant.

Premature menopause

The fixed pool of primordial oocytes in the human ovary declines with increasing age until the menopause is reached at around 50–51 years. The age of onset of the menopause varies between individual women and is marked by the final menstrual cycle when the primordial ovarian follicles are exhausted. Decline in fertility begins well before the menopause. The rate of follicle decline is steady from puberty to about the age of 37 years when about 25 000 follicles remain. Subsequently the rate of loss of follicles increases, with the menopause occurring about 12–14 years later. It has been estimated that only about 1000 primordial follicles may remain at menopause. As around only 400 ovulations occur in a reproductive lifetime, the huge loss of follicles is attributed to a process of apoptosis (programmed cell death), rather than ovulation. Premature excessive loss of oocytes leads to premature menopause in about 2% of teenagers and women in their early 20s.

For young women who have undergone menopause, and want a baby, the only treatment option is *in vitro* fertilization of a donated egg by the partner's sperm followed by transfer of embryo into the uterus. The egg donor undergoes the treatment cycle for inducing multiple follicular development (Figure 4.15). In the meantime, the recipient is given oestrogen for 2 weeks before embryo transfer, in order to stimulate development of her uterine lining so that it is ready to receive an implanting embryo. The donor's oocytes are harvested, and are fertilized *in vitro* with the recipient's partner's sperm. The embryos are allowed to develop for 5–6 days, to the blastocyst stage. On the day before blastocyst transfer, progesterone is administered to the recipient. Oestrogen and progesterone treatment are continued in the recipient, and a pregnancy test carried out 8 days after embryo transfer. If pregnancy is confirmed, oestrogen and progesterone treatment are continued for 10 weeks.

As we have seen, there are treatment options for female infertility and these can provide a good outcome, a healthy baby, for a high proportion of cases. In contrast, as we shall see in the following section, male infertility is more difficult to treat.

Summary of Section 4.5

1   Female infertility due to blocked fallopian tubes can be detected by hysterosalpingography, in which a radio-opaque dye is infused into the uterus. Leakage of dye into the abdominal cavity indicates open tubes; dye remaining in the uterus indicates blocked tubes.

2   Blocked fallopian tubes are caused by scarring and adhesions resulting from infections such as chlamydia and gonorrhea that cause pelvic inflammatory disease, PID. If surgery to clear tubes is ineffective, *in vitro* fertilization is recommended.

3   Oocytes are harvested for IVF following shut-down of the woman's own menstrual cycle by a GnRH analogue and is controlled subsequently by FSH injections. Persistent high blood FSH levels stimulate growth and maturation of up to around 10 follicles in the ovaries.

4   Disorders of ovulation may be treated by administration of clomiphene citrate, which stimulates FSH secretion by the pituitary. There is a risk of hyperstimulation of the ovary.

5   Polycystic ovarian syndrome (PCOS) is characterized by ovaries with many cysts, and small follicles, which produce large amounts of testosterone. Ovulation may be absent or sporadic. Fertility treatment may be successful.

6   Infertility due to premature menopause can be overcome by IVF using donated eggs. The infertile recipient of the embryos takes oestrogen and progesterone to prepare her uterus for implantation of the embryo.

4.6 Low sperm counts, and infertility in men

Sperm counts in fertile men are in the range of $50–150 \times 10^6$ sperm ml^{-1} (Table 4.1) and at least 60% of the sperm fully motile. Disorders in sperm production and sperm function are a major cause of difficulty in conceiving, accounting for 25% of infertility in couples. Male infertility derives from either low sperm counts, known as **oligospermia**, or no sperm at all, known as **aspermia**. Absence of sperm or low sperm counts may be a result of blocked transport of sperm from seminiferous tubules or may derive from deficient production. Oligospermia is often associated with various sperm defects including reduced motility, abnormal morphologies and genetic defects.

Table 4.1 World Health Organization criteria for 'normal' and 'subfertile' semen (Johnson and Everitt, 2000, adapted from WHO, 1992).

Criterion	Normal	Subfertile
Volume in a typical ejaculate/ml	2–5	1
Sperm concentration/number ml^{-1} semen	$50–150 \times 10^6$	$< 20 \times 10^6$
Total sperm number in an ejaculate	$100–700 \times 10^6$	$< 50 \times 10^6$
Spermatozoa swimming forward vigorously/%	$> 60\%$	$< 40\%$
Abnormal spermatozoa/%	$< 30\%$	$> 60\%$
Viscosity after liquefaction	Low	High
Cellular debris, leukocytes and immature sperm cells	Low but variable	High

Low sperm counts are associated with smaller testes than normal, generally less than 20 ml in volume and of a softer consistency than normal. A study of semen quality is always carried out during investigation of the cause of infertility in a couple. Semen may be obtained from an ejaculate, or recovered post-coitally from the cervix. Defective endocrine control of spermatogenesis as a cause of male infertility is rare; in such cases treatment with GnRH or gonadotropins may be successful (Section 4.2.1).

4.6.1 Causal factors linked to aspermia and oligospermia

Temporary oligospermia can be caused by controllable factors, including dietary deficiency, for example, insufficient essential fatty acids, vitamins B$_{12}$, C and E and zinc (Book 1 Sections 3.4 and 3.7). Exposure to X-ray irradiation and excessive alcohol intake are also factors that contribute to declining sperm counts. Increased scrotal temperature due to tight-fitting underwear or frequent long hot baths may reduce sperm count. Dietary deficiency and excessive alcohol intake can be corrected, and loose-fitting underwear worn to prevent over-heating of the testes. Hot baths can be avoided and warm, not hot, showers should be the norm. Exposure to X-ray irradiation at work or during cancer treatment can be minimized by appropriate precautions, such as the use of lead shielding.

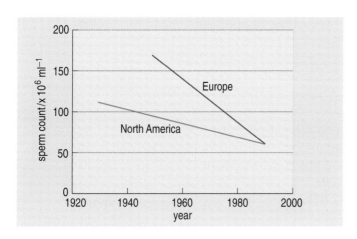

Figure 4.17 Mean sperm counts derived from compilation of data from various studies in North America and Europe (Sharpe and Irvine, 2004).

A number of scientists and clinicians have expressed concern that male fertility is declining.

● Examine the data in Figure 4.17, and describe the main trends quoting values from the data to support your description.

◐ There is a sharp decline in sperm count from the late 1950s to 1990 in Europe and a slow decline from 1930 to 1990 in North America. Sperm counts declined from $> 150 \times 10^6$ sperm ml^{-1} in 1950 in Europe to about 60×10^6 sperm ml^{-1} in 1990. In North America sperm counts declined from 120×10^6 ml^{-1} in 1958 to 60×10^6 sperm ml^{-1} in 1995.

● Study the data in Table 4.1. Are the decreased sperm counts indicated in Figure 4.17 likely to be linked to decreased fertility?

◐ It is unlikely that the decline in sperm counts indicated in Figure 4.17 would be noticed as a decrease in fertility as even the lowest values are still within the range for 'normal' fertility quoted in Table 4.1.

Chemical pollutants in the environment have been blamed for a decrease in sperm count over the last 50–60 years. Attention has focused on environmental pollutants that mimic oestrogens, especially *phthalates*, chemicals used in plastics manufacture, and also in vinyl flooring, paints and inks. A study of 168 men, of average age 34.6 years, who were attending a fertility clinic at Massachusetts General Hospital in the USA, involved carrying out a sperm count for each man and analysing their urine samples for derivatives of phthalate (Duty et al., 2003). Measurements carried out on the semen samples were sperm concentration, motility and criteria for normal appearance. Urine analyses identified five different phthalate-derived compounds. Overall 54% of the men had measured sperm characteristics lower than at least one of the World Health Organization's criteria for 'normal' semen (Table 4.1).

The researchers identified one of the phthalate-derived chemicals, mono-n-butylphthalate (MBP), as being particularly important. Men with high levels of urinary MBP were more than twice as likely to have low sperm motility and low sperm count. Nearly twice as many of the men with high urinary MBP levels had deformed sperm in comparison with the men without MBP in their urine.

● Suggest reasons other than phthalate pollution for low sperm counts and decreased sperm motility in the men attending the fertility clinic.

● Sperm counts can also be decreased by other factors, e.g. dietary deficiency, high alcohol intake.

The men attending the fertility clinic may also not be representative of the population, so caution is required in interpreting the findings. However, studies such as that carried out on the men at Massachusetts General Hospital have indicated higher levels of human exposure to phthalates than had been realized before. Whether the sperm count and sperm motility of the men would recover after clearance of phthalate from the body or whether the effect is permanent is not known.

One irreversible cause of low sperm counts is insufficient spermatogenesis caused by undescended testes. Usually the testes, which develop in the abdominal cavity, descend into the scrotum shortly before birth. In a few baby boys the testes do not descend until around 4 months after birth. If the testes have still not descended by 6 months, surgery is required to place the testes in the scrotum. As this is done routinely in most parts of the world undescended testes are now an unlikely cause of male infertility.

Genetic abnormalities including Klinefelter's syndrome may account for oligospermia and aspermia.

● What is the sexual genotype for Klineflelter's syndrome, and the associated signs?

● Men with Klinefelter's syndrome have genotype XXY and are healthy, but they may be unaware of their aspermia (Case Report 1.2). During childhood there may be difficulties in language development that affect reading and writing ability.

Certain infections can result in temporary or permanent aspermia or oligospermia. Inflammation of the testes (orchitis) may be a consequence of infection with the mumps virus or bacterial infections such as chlamydia, gonorrhea, syphilis or tuberculosis. Epididymo-orchitis is bacterial inflammation of testes and epididymis and may be caused by urinary infections, gonorrhea and tuberculosis, or may be idiopathic.

● Suggest an explanation for aspermia caused by epididymo-orchitis.

● The epididymis consists of many small tubules (Figure 4.1), through which the spermatozoa pass before being transferred into the vas deferens. Infections of the epididymis may cause blockage of these tubules.

Damage caused to the tubules in the epididymis by the infection may result in permanent obstructive aspermia and infertility. Surgery that attempts to bypass the epididymal tubules has been unsuccessful in restoring fertility.

● Why would spermatozoa that bypass the epididymis be incapable of fertilization?

● While spermatozoa are in the epididymis, they are coated with glycoproteins, and nourished by sugary secretions (Section 4.2.1), which are essential for swimming ability.

High levels of sluggish or dead sperm in the ejaculate suggest sub-optimal spermatogenesis and may be due to genetic abnormalities, infections of the genital tract and antisperm antibodies in testicular fluids. Treatments for intransigent male infertility are based on variants of IVF, as we shall see in the following section.

4.6.2 Treatment of male infertility

Where the ejaculate contains at least some healthy spermatozoa, these can be isolated from dead and damaged ones and concentrated so that a relatively high concentration of healthy sperm can be mixed with oocytes in a dish for *in vitro* fertilization (Figure 4.18a). After collection of an ejaculate for IVF, the spermatozoa are examined with a microscope to assess their quality. Dead or sluggish sperm and those that appear abnormal can be separated from viable healthy motile sperm.

Capacitation of the sperm (Section 4.3.3) is achieved *in vitro* by washing the sperm in suitable fluids. The sperm sample is then ready for adding to the dish containing the woman's oocytes. Sperm and oocytes may then be mixed and transferred by laparoscopy into the fallopian tube where fertilization occurs. This procedure is known as gamete intrafallopian transfer (GIFT).

When sperm counts are very low, *in vitro* fertilization may be accomplished by drilling a small hole in the zona pellucida, a procedure known as zonal drilling (ZD) (Figure 4.20b), which facilitates sperm entry.

Two techniques of IVF may be used where sperm numbers are even lower. In subzonal insemination (SUZI), sperm are injected underneath the zona (Figure 4.18c). ICSI, intracytoplasmic injection of a single sperm cell into an oocyte (Figure 4.18d), can be used where there are no motile spermatozoa or even where only testicular spermatozoa are available, as in obstructive aspermia. Spermatozoa extracted from the epididymis or testis can be used for SUZI or ICSI (Figure 4.19). Each sperm is examined very carefully to ensure that it has normal structure before injection into an oocyte.

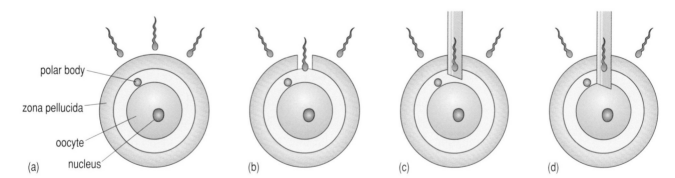

Figure 4.18 Techniques of *in vitro* fertilization that are used to treat infertility. (a) For IVF, oocytes are collected from the female partner's ovary or from an egg donor's ovary after stimulation with FSH. Spermatozoa are collected from the male partner or from a donor male. Oocytes and sperm are then mixed in the dish for 24–48 hours. (b) Zonal drilling (ZD) is the same as IVF but before insemination a hole is drilled in the zona pellucida by laser or application of a zona-dissolving chemical, which facilitates entry of sperm. (c) Subzonal insemination (SUZI) involves placing one or more spermatozoa beneath the zona using a micropipette. (d) Intracytoplasmic injection (ICSI) involves use of a micropipette to inject a single sperm cell into the cytoplasm of the oocyte. Fertilized oocytes can be identified by the appearance of pronuclei and cleavage into two to four cells.

● Both SUZI and ICSI are controversial, so much so that one view demands that these procedures be banned. Suggest the reason for the controversy. *Hint*: re-read Section 4.6.1, which outlines the causes of male infertility.

● As some oligospermic conditions have a genetic cause it is possible that SUZI and ICSI will pass on the oligospermia to male offspring.

The concern is justified in part, as some cases of obstructive aspermia are found in men who have just one copy of the allele for cystic fibrosis (CF) and are otherwise asymptomatic. There is a risk that use of SUZI or ICSI will pass the CF gene to offspring.

Having considered the problem of infertility in men and women, we now move on to the situation where there is an embryo ready to implant in the uterus, as we left it at the end of Section 4.3.

Summary of Section 4.6

1 Oligospermia and aspermia are significant causes of infertility in couples.

2 Temporary aspermia may be caused by controllable factors such as dietary deficiency or excessive alcohol intake and can be corrected.

3 There is evidence that environmental pollution, especially by chemicals that are similar to oestrogens, e.g. phthalates, can cause low sperm counts.

4 Irreversible aspermia can be caused by genetic abnormalities such as Klinefelter's syndrome, or tubular blockage in the epididymis resulting from infections.

5 IVF can be used to overcome male infertility where sperm counts are low. Sperm of normal appearance and motility are collected from a sperm sample, concentrated and added to a dish containing oocytes for IVF. A hole may be drilled in the zona (zonal drilling, ZD) of oocytes to facilitate sperm penetration.

6 Special techniques of IVF are used for aspermia, in which sperm can be collected from the testis or epididymis. In subzonal drilling, SUZI, sperm are injected beneath the zona. For ICSI, intracytoplasmic injection, a single sperm cell is injected into oocyte cytoplasm.

4.7 A healthy embryo

Every pregnant woman longs for a healthy baby and fortunately most babies are indeed healthy. There is much that a woman can do herself to provide for the nutritional needs of her developing baby, and to protect her embryo and fetus from noxious and toxic substances such as cigarettes and alcohol. GPs and health visitors at antenatal clinics provide leaflets with information about nutrition and with advice for women who are planning a pregnancy or who are in the very early stages of pregnancy.

During pregnancy, a woman can meet the nutritional needs of the developing fetus by eating a healthy diet (Book 1, Figure 3.1). Carbohydrates such as wholemeal bread, chapattis, rice, pasta, couscous, breakfast cereal, and potatoes should make up about a third of the food intake. These foods provide energy and fibre too. Wholemeal breads and cereals also contain folic acid, an essential vitamin for the developing fetus.

- Why is it important for both pregnant mother and developing fetus to have adequate folic acid? *Hint*: refer to Book 1, Chapter 3 if necessary.

- Folic acid is essential for DNA synthesis, so rapidly proliferating cells such as stem cells in bone marrow are affected by folic acid deficiency which can result in megaloblastic anaemia in pregnant women. Folic acid is also important for the fetus as it has been shown to reduce the incidence of spina bifida (Book 1, Section 3.7.2).

Fruits and vegetables are recommended to make up another third of the diet and they can provide iron (leafy vegetables) and vitamins C and A (e.g. apples, bananas, carrots, mangoes, peppers) and folic acid (potatoes, green vegetables, oranges). Meat, fish and pulses contain protein and iron. Milk, yoghurt and cheeses provide protein.

- Dairy products are recommended as being an essential part of the diet for a pregnant woman. What mineral nutrient is provided by dairy products, and why is it essential for the developing fetus?

- Dairy products such as milk, yoghurt and cheese contain calcium, important for building the skeleton of the developing fetus.

- Is the following statement true or false? Explain your reasoning. 'A pregnant mother should be eating for two, so pregnancy is a time when you can enjoy all your favourite chocolate bars, biscuits, crisps and cakes'.

- False. An increased intake of 200 kcal per day is required in the final 3 months of pregnancy (Book 1, Table 3.1) and can be met by eating more carbohydrates, fruit and vegetables. Increasing intake of fatty and sugary foods such as cakes, crisps, biscuits and chocolate bars would not be recommended. These foods should make up the smallest fraction of the diet, as they have low vitamin and essential nutrient content, and their high energy (fat) content places consumers at risk of obesity.

Pregnant women are advised to avoid cheeses made from unpasteurized milk, because of the risk of food poisoning, in particular by the bacterium *Listeria*, which can cause miscarriage.

Research studies suggest a link between high caffeine consumption and miscarriage so it is recommended that caffeine intake should be limited to less than 300 mg per day. This amount of caffeine would be contained in three cups of coffee or six cups of tea. Women trying to conceive or who are pregnant are advised to avoid drinking alcohol, or at least to limit intake to one or two units (one or two glasses of wine) per week. Serious effects of fetal exposure to alcohol are seen in babies born to mothers who drink large quantities of alcohol throughout pregnancy. Fetal alcohol syndrome is the extreme result of alcohol abuse during pregnancy. Affected babies have nervous system problems, impaired growth and abnormal facial features such as small eye openings. Long-term effects include behavioural and functional problems. Evidence from experiments on mice suggests that exposure to alcohol or smoking around the time of ovulation and fertilization can disrupt the complex processes of meiosis, fertilization, and cleavage of the embryo. Embryos derived by IVF of oocytes from female mice who were given water containing 10% ethanol for 30 days showed a higher rate of abnormalities than did embryos from the control group of female mice given water containing the sugars maltose and dextrin. Abnormalities in the embryos from the alcohol-treated mice included fragmentation, cells of unequal size, and lack of cleavage division with signs of cell death. By day 5, when most embryos from the control mice were at the blastocyst stage, very few embryos from the alcohol-treated mothers had reached the blastocyst stage (Cebral et al., 1999).

Certain medicines and pollutants, known as **teratogens**, can affect development of the fetus. The thalidomide tragedy in the 1960s highlighted the dangers. Thalidomide was prescribed to counteract nausea and aid sleep in early pregnancy but when taken at 39–42 days after conception, it caused malformations of the limbs such as lack of arms and legs because it inhibited proliferation of cells that would have formed parts of the limbs. Since the thalidomide tragedy, more stringent tests are made on the drugs prescribed for use in pregnancy, and current advice is that only medicines prescribed by a doctor should be taken by women who are pregnant or trying to conceive. Ibuprofen, a popular pain killer, is not recommended for women in the third trimester of pregnancy as studies suggest that it may cause premature closure of the ductus arteriosus (a blood vessel in the fetal heart) which can cause high blood pressure in the fetal lungs (OTIS, 2004).

Smoking is dangerous for the developing fetus at all stages of development and the advice to pregnant women is to avoid smoking and also to avoid spending time in areas where other people are smoking. Exposure of the developing fetus to smoke causes increased risk of miscarriage, and also low birth weight.

There are also factors that we cannot control which affect the health of babies and we examine these in the following section.

4.7.1 Chromosome abnormalities and mutation

Recall from Chapter 1 that the process of recombination during meiosis has a huge impact on us.

● Meiosis halves the number of chromosomes during gametogenesis. How does this type of cell division result in variability and what does this imply for offspring?

● Meiosis reshuffles the maternal and paternal alleles resulting in new combinations of alleles (Figure 1.5c–e), providing a major source of variation in human populations (Section 1.2.2). So a child born to a couple may bear little resemblance to either parent, because particular combinations of alleles were lost in chromosome shuffling during meiosis.

Variation derived from meiosis is advantageous for us (Section 1.2.4) and yet there is a cost, in that chromosome abnormalities may arise in sperm and oocytes. Aneuploidies, in which there is either an extra chromosome or a chromosome is missing, are the most common chromosome abnormalities in human embryos (Table 1.1 and Figure 1.6). Most embryos with chromosome aneuploidies are lost at early stages of development. However, a few aneuploidies are compatible with survival, e.g. trisomy of chromosome 21 which causes Down's syndrome.

Structural rearrangements of chromosomes happen when a piece of a chromosome breaks off and then becomes attached to another chromosome. Some rearrangements cause no problems and there is a high survival rate for affected embryos (Table 1.1). Certain chromosome rearrangements cause serious problems. For example, *Prader–Willi syndrome* results from structural rearrangements in chromosome 15, usually a small deletion in the paternal chromosome. Affected neonates have low birth weight, poor muscle tone, and they are reluctant feeders. However, between the ages of 2 and 4 the children switch to having an insatiable appetite for food, which can lead to lethal obesity. The children have short stature and behavioural problems. Treatment regimens are demanding for carers, as life-long care is required, including strict monitoring of food intake.

The only source of genetic variation that is heritable is spontaneous gene mutation (Section 1.2.1). Some mutations have little effect and cause no harm and no particular benefit. For example, some types of heritable polydactyly, extra fingers or toes, have no other associated signs, and can be treated by simple removal of the extra digits. Other mutations cause serious or lethal disease (Table 4.2) but they are rare. Diagnosis of a genetic disorder such as cystic fibrosis or Tay–Sachs disease in a baby is devastating news for the family, compounded by concerns about transmission of that disorder to other offspring. Inevitably the entire extended family is involved as all members have a shared genetic inheritance.

Genetic counsellors help families to come to terms with diagnoses of genetic disease in a baby, and they keep up to date with developments in treatment and prevention. In this way the parents of the child are provided with the information they need, including the risk of transmission to future offspring and availability of new treatments. Babies identified as having cystic fibrosis, for example, will begin a lifetime programme of treatment including physiotherapy, enzyme supplements

Table 4.2   Examples of human genetic diseases.

Genetic disease and incidence	Signs and symptoms	Compatibility with life
Cystic fibrosis Incidence: c. 0.4 in 1000 births in the UK	Sticky mucus affects lung function; enzyme secretion by pancreas blocked, preventing digestion	With treatment, e.g. physiotherapy for clearing lung mucus, patients are surviving to their fourth decade
Tay–Sachs disease Mean incidence: c. 1 in 300 000; higher in Ashkenazi Jewish people	Degeneration of brain begins at 6 months; blindness and excessive muscle tone result	Affected children live for up to 4 years; cause of death is usually lung infection
Duchenne muscular dystrophy; caused by a mutation on the X chromosome Incidence: c. 0.3 in 1000 births in the UK	Only boys are affected as the Y chromosome cannot mask the effects of the mutant gene in the X chromosome Muscle wasting, frequent falls and waddling gait appear in first 5 years of life	Patients are usually unable to walk by age 10, and need a wheelchair. Death occurs by the age of 20–30 years when breathing is prevented by paralysis of the intercostal and diaphragm muscles
Huntington's disease; caused by a gene mutation Incidence: c. 0.5 in 1000 births in the UK	Brain deterioration begins in middle age, expressed as forgetfulness, mood swings, clumsiness, progressing to involuntary movements and difficulty in swallowing	Once symptoms appear, progression to requiring full nursing care takes up to 20 years Death often results from pneumonia

and for some patients, heart and lung transplants. These provide a life expectancy of about 30–40 years in contrast to just 10 years in the 1960s.

Genetic mutations and the high incidence of chromosome abnormalities in gametes have an impact on the success rates of IVF. If high proportions of apparently healthy embryos produced by IVF have chromosome abnormalities, few embryos transferred develop into a successful pregnancy. In the following section we see how research at IVF clinics led to the development of tests for detection of genetic diseases and chromosome abnormalities at very early stages of development of the embryo.

4.7.2 Pre-implantation genetic diagnosis and screening

Parents having a child with a genetic disease such as cystic fibrosis, who are not affected themselves, each carry one copy of the mutant gene. They therefore have a one in four chance of having another affected child with two copies of the gene and a one in four chance of having a baby who carries no mutant gene at all. In the early 1990s, IVF clinics devised a technique for pre-implantation genetic diagnosis, PGD, in which one or two cells are removed from each eight-celled embryo produced by IVF. Normal development continues in the embryos after removal of the cells.

Tests are carried out on the cells removed from the embryos to determine whether they have genes coding for genetic diseases. Embryos that carry no mutant genes are used for transfer to the woman. Initially PGD was used to screen for embryos carrying mutations that cause serious genetic diseases including Duchenne muscular dystrophy, Tay–Sachs disease and cystic fibrosis; by 2004 all the most common serious genetic conditions were included. Parents who have already had a child with a serious genetic disease may opt for IVF with PGD in order to have a healthy embryo identified. Costs are high, around £6000 (in 2005), but considered worthwhile by many couples, for a chance to have a healthy baby. Two hundred children born after PGD carried out in various European clinics are being followed up by a group of researchers including Alan Handyside (Leeds University) (Westphal, 2004). So far the results are looking positive.

A similar technique, pre-implantation genetic screening (PGS), is used to identify chromosome abnormalities such as aneuploidy and chromosome structural rearrangements. DNA probes are attached to different coloured fluorescent dyes, which light up when they link to particular chromosomes. Figure 4.19 shows how an extra chromosome 18, coloured blue, was revealed in a nucleus from a cell in a female 8-cell embryo.

- Why is PGS particularly helpful for women aged > 40 years who want to have a baby by IVF?

- As the incidence of aneuploidy in oocytes increases sharply beyond maternal age of 40 years, PGS increases the chances of a healthy embryo and baby for older mothers (Section 1.2.3).

Currently early PGS (2005) looks at 10 of the 24 different human chromosomes but research is focusing on extending the test to all the chromosomes. By ensuring that only healthy embryos are transferred, PGD increases the chances of a

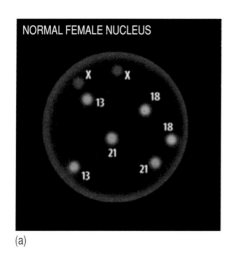

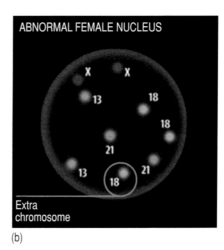

(a)   (b)

Figure 4.19 Results of a PGD screening for chromosomal abnormalities. After a cell is removed from an embryo special fluorescent dyes are used that attach to particular chromosomes. In this case three chromosome 18s, coloured blue, were revealed.

woman having a healthy baby. Increasing numbers of couples are opting for IVF with PGS, even though the cost per treatment cycle in 2005 is close to £5000.

4.7.3 A healthy baby

In this chapter we have not examined development of the embryo beyond the blastocyst stage. Now we jump ahead and look briefly at how during late pregnancy fetal physiological systems develop and mature in preparation for life outside the uterus. For example, changes in the fetal lung prepare the way for breathing air. From about 7 months of pregnancy lung surfactant appears, which reduces the surface tension of the lungs (Book 3, Section 3.2.1) and helps the baby to take the first breath after birth. In the uterus, the fetus makes rapid respiratory movements that move amniotic fluid in and out of the lungs. Such movements distend the lungs and may help to promote their growth. During a vaginal delivery, fluid in the baby's lungs is lost through the mouth and any remaining fluid is resorbed. Normal breathing begins quickly and gaseous exchange is established. At the same time birth brings about major changes in the baby's blood circulatory system. When in the uterus, the fetal blood is diverted away from the lungs to the placenta where gas exchange occurs. This is accomplished by two vascular shunts (Book 3, Section 2.3.2). One of these shunts, the *foramen ovale,* diverts blood from the right atrium of the heart into the left ventricle by-passing the right ventricle. Much of the blood that does go to the right ventricle is diverted by the *ductus arteriosus* into the aorta, thereby also by-passing the lungs. During birth, when blood circulation to placenta is cut off by severance of the umbilical cord, the three shunts are closed, so that blood starts to circulate through the lungs. The respiratory and blood vascular systems of a new-born baby therefore adapt rapidly to air-breathing.

However, a difficult prolonged labour can cause harm to even a healthy baby, in particular if the baby has been starved of oxygen for a long time. Therefore the health status of a new-born baby is monitored very soon after birth, using the 'Apgar score,' which was devised by Dr Virginia Apgar (1953). When a new baby is born, the time is noted, and the Apgar score is determined at precisely one minute and five minutes after birth (Table 4.3). The criteria listed for scores of 2 define features of a healthy new-born baby, but cannot be used to predict the long-term health of the baby.

Table 4.3   Criteria used for assessment of Apgar score in new-born babies.

Score	0	1	2
Heart rate/beats min^{-1}	Absent	< 100	> 100
Respirations	Absent	Slow or irregular breaths	Regular strong breaths with strong cry
Muscle tone	Limp	Some flexion of arms and legs	Active motion
Reflex irritability*	Absent	Grimace	Grimace and vigorous cough and sneeze
Colour (whole body or mouth and palms of hands and feet)	Blue or pale	Pink body with blue hands and feet	Completely pink

*Reaction to pinching nose.

A total score of < 7 or 7 at one minute suggests a baby may have had problems during labour that reduced the oxygen in the blood. It may be necessary to clear the baby's airways. Babies with Apgar scores of 4 or less may need oxygen and special care. However, most babies with lower Apgar scores at 1 minute, have normal oxygen levels and become more active later. If further intervention is required the Apgar score is measured at 5-minute intervals until the score is at least 6. The Apgar score is helpful as it enables midwives to determine quickly whether a new-born baby needs help, and at the 5-minute stage, to monitor the effects of any help that was provided. Monitoring new-born babies in this way helps to ensure that babies stay healthy.

Summary of Section 4.7

1   During pregnancy a healthy diet and avoidance of alcohol, smoking, unprescribed drugs and environmental pollution help to increase the chances of having a healthy baby.

2   As most chromosome abnormalities and genetic mutations are incompatible with embryonic development most new-born babies are healthy. Severe genetic diseases are rare.

3   Following IVF pre-implantation screening and genetic diagnosis can be used to identify healthy embryos for transfer to a recipient.

4   Healthy embryos are likely to develop into healthy babies and in late pregnancy maturational changes in lungs prepare the fetus for breathing air. Closure of vascular shunts in the blood circulation system divert a new-born baby's blood circulation to the lungs.

5   Careful monitoring of new-born babies using the Apgar score identifies those with difficulties, e.g. in obtaining oxygen, so measures can be taken to help them, and to keep them healthy.

4.8 Conclusion

In this chapter we have examined how we can produce healthy babies. Healthy babies have viable phenotypes, derived from gametes with viable genotypes. Meiosis, the pivotal process in gametogenesis involves not just production of gametes, but also a re-shuffling of maternal and paternal genotypes. Fertilization is random; any one of a huge variety of sperm could be the one that fertilizes an oocyte. As the genotypes of oocytes have a similar degree of variability to those of sperm, fertilization results in even more variation in the zygote!

Genetic variation in humans has a cost in that gene mutations or errors in meiosis result in serious or lethal consequences for the developing embryo. Yet this variation contributed to the ability of our species to colonize and live successfully in a huge variety of climates and social conditions. Although most of us now live in towns or cities, we are not isolated from environmental factors that can affect our survival. In a busy city environment, for example, individuals who can cope with stress may be those most likely to produce healthy offspring. We saw in Chapter 1 that embryos with variations that are incompatible with life are lost at very early stages of development, a process which increases our chances of having a healthy baby. Couples who are infertile can be helped to have a healthy baby by treatments available at fertility clinics. Recent development of pre-implantation diagnosis and screening increase the chances that the embryos transferred to a recipient are healthy. Pregnant women can do much to maintain the health of their developing fetus by eating a suitable diet and avoiding alcohol, smoking and non-prescription drug treatments.

Many babies who are born with a health problem can be treated successfully. New treatment regimens devised for certain genetic and chromosomal diseases have prolonged life and improved quality of life for affected babies. Even for some of those conditions where treatment is not yet available, research is making progress. However, in certain cases where a baby is born with untreatable abnormalities incompatible with life, all that can be done is to make the short life of the baby, even if just a few hours, as comfortable as possible with maximum contact with the parents.

So while we have to accept the reality that a small proportion of babies are born with untreatable health problems, the good news is that most babies are healthy and happy (Figure 4.20).

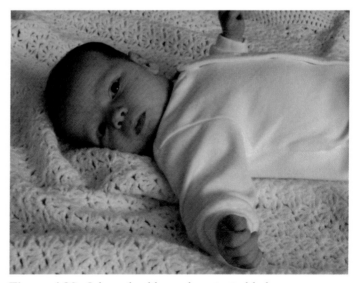

Figure 4.20 Jobe, a healthy and contented baby.

Questions for Chapter 4

Question 4.1 (LOs 4.1–4.3)

Classify the following as true, partly true or false, and explain your view for each.

(a) The hypothalamic–pituitary axis is involved in the control of both spermatogenesis and oogenesis.

(b) Oogenesis is cyclic but spermatogenesis is not.

(c) Spermatogenesis can continue throughout a man's life whereas in women, oogenesis ceases around the age of 50–55.

(d) Sex steroids exert negative feedback on the anterior pituitary in both males and females.

(e) The epididymis is simply a storage area for mature spermatozoa from where they are released into the vas deferens.

(f) Fertilization comprises the instant fusion of a sperm cell with an oocyte.

Question 4.2 (LOs 4.1–4.3)

Study Figures 4.2, 4.3 and 4.5 and summarize the stages of spermatogenesis and their location as a set of bullet points.

Question 4.3 (LO 4.2)

Examine Figure 4.21 carefully, and answer the following questions:

(i) Describe the levels of LH and FSH in each of (a) and (b) and identify the main comparisons that you can make.

(ii) Explain the different patterns in (a) and (b) with reference to the role of the hypothalamic–pituitary axis in controlling the cycle.

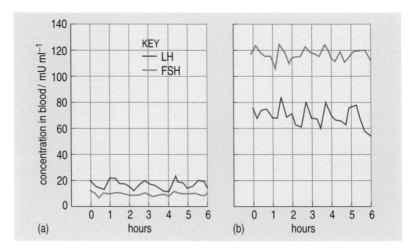

Figure 4.21 Level of circulating LH (red) and FSH (blue) (arbitrary units) in: (a) a woman at day 8 in the early follicular phase; and (b) a post-menopausal woman.

Question 4.4 (LOs 4.1, 4.2 and 4.4)

Explain why taking combined oral contraceptive pills (COCs) suppresses follicular growth and development and secretion of oestrogens by the ovary.

Question 4.5 (LOs 4.2, 4.3, 4.8)

Suggest an explanation for the observation that hCG may be detected during a prolonged late luteal phase of the menstrual cycle, i.e. at about 18–30 days after the last menstrual period, but there is no pregnancy detected later.

Question 4.6 (LOs 4.2 and 4.6)

A couple in their late thirties have been trying for a baby for 8 years but no pregnancy has resulted. The husband Michael, aged 37, has a normal sperm count with < 20% abnormal sperm, and the wife Jane, aged 39 years, has irregular menstrual cycles. After two failed IVF treatment cycles, their consultant suggests egg donation, and IVF of the donated eggs using Michael's sperm.

Drawing on information in Table 4.1, and Section 4.3, outline the rationale for the hormonal treatment that is likely to be administered to Jane, the recipient of the embryo. The embryo, as is usual for those created from donor eggs, is transferred at the blastocyst stage, 6 days after fertilization.

Question 4.7 (LOs 4.7 and 4.8)

Siegfried, aged 35, and his wife Maria aged 27, years have been unsuccessful in achieving pregnancy after 3 years of trying. Tests at a fertility clinic reveal that Siegfried has no sperm at all. Maria has normal menstrual cycles and no fallopian tube blockages. (i) Suggest the options for fertility treatment that a clinic might recommend. (ii) What would clinicians at the fertility clinic want to know about Siegfried's genetic history before proceeding with any of the treatments? Explain your answer with reference to infertility treatment and possible further tests.

References

Apgar, V. (1953) A proposal for a new method of evaluation for the new-born infant. *Current Researches in Anaesthesia and Analgesia*, **32**, 260–267.

Cebral, E., Lasserre, A., Rettori, V. and de Gimeno, M.A. (1999) Deleterious effects of moderate alcohol intake by female mice on pre-implantation embryo growth *in vitro*. *Alcohol and Alcoholism*, **34**, 551–558.

Christiansen, P. and Skakkebaek, N. E. (2002) Pulsatile gonadotropin-releasing hormone treatment of men with idiopathic hypogonadotropic hypogonadism. *Hormone Research*, **57**, 32–36.

Duty, S. M., Silva, M. J., Barr, D. B., Brock, J. W., Ryan, L., Chen, Z., Herrick, R.F., Christiani, D. C. and Hauser, R. (2003) Phthalate exposure and human semen parameters. *Epidemiology*, **14**, 269–277.

Gomes, M. P. and Deitcher, S. R. (2004) Risks of venous thromboembolic disease associated with hormonal contraceptives and hormone replacement therapy: a clinical review. *Archives of Internal Medicine*, **164**, 1965–1976.

Jaiswal, B. J., Tur-Kaspa, I., Dor, J., Mashiach, S. and Eisenbach, M. (1999) Human sperm chemotaxis: is progesterone a chemoattractant? *Biology of Reproduction*, **69**, 1314–1319.

Johnson, M. H. and Everitt, B. J. (2000) *Essential Reproduction*, 5th edn. Oxford: Blackwell Science.

OTIS: Organization of Teratology Information Services (2004) [online] Fact Sheets: Caffeine and Pregnancy; Ibuprofen and Pregnancy. Available from: www.OTISpregnancy.org (Accessed February 2005)

Multiple Births Foundation (2004) Queen Charlotte's and Chelsea Hospital, West London [online]. Available from: http://www.multiplebirths.org.uk/index.asp (Accessed February 2005)

Practical Support for Clinical Governance PRODIGY (2004) Pelvic Inflammatory Disease [online]. Available from: http://www.prodigy.nhs.uk/ guidance.asp?gt=Pelvic%20inflammatory%20disease (Accessed February 2005)

Sharpe, R. M. and Irvine, D. S. (2004) How strong is the evidence of a link between environmental chemicals and adverse effects on human reproductive health? *British Medical Journal*, **328**, 447–451.

Victory, R., D'Souza, C., Diamond, M. P., McNeeley, S. G., Vista-Deck, D. and Hendrix, S. (2004) Adverse cardiovascular outcomes are reduced in women with a history of oral contraceptive use: Results from the Women's Health Initiative database. *Fertility and Sterility*, **82**, S52–S53.

Westphal, S. P. (2004) The rush to pick a perfect embryo. *New Scientist*, **182**, 6–7.

World Health Organization (1992) *Laboratory Manual for the Examination of Human Semen and Sperm-cervical Mucus Interaction*, 3rd edn. Cambridge: Cambridge University Press

World Health Organization (2004) Current Practices and Controversies in Assisted Reproduction [online]. Available from: http://www.who.int/reproductive-health/infertility/index.htm (Accessed February 2005)

ANSWERS TO QUESTIONS

Question 1.1

Increased body weight is likely to result in increased numbers and changed function in the cells that make up adipose tissue. But there is no obvious mechanism through which these changes are likely to affect the genetic constitution of the cells in the ovaries or testes that give rise to eggs or sperm and which are laid down early in development. In the same way, if you take up body-building you will not make it more likely that you have muscular children unless you plan to pay for their gym subscriptions as well!

Question 1.2

Point mutations will change, at the most, only a single amino acid within the resulting protein. Sometimes such a change will have little effect on the function of this protein. (It may have no effect at all.) However, if the changed amino acid is at a critical point, perhaps where a neurotransmitter binds to a protein receptor, it may cause more serious disruption. By contrast the effects of a frame shift mutation are not restricted to a single site, but cascade down the resulting amino acid chain. Movement of a gene, or group of genes, from one chromosome to another can also have very serious effects because it may disrupt the mechanisms that switch gene expression on and off.

Question 1.3

By now you should realize that it is very hard to answer this question for any particular person. Certainly the case report does not give the necessary information, although it does suggest some possible factors, such as increased food intake, that are more likely than others. But, in general, even strong trends and associations at the population level, do not provide unambiguous explanations at the levels of individuals.

Question 1.4

Bray's analogy is memorable and for the specific point he is making it does ring true. However it implies a definite order; load gun; pull trigger and one outcome; bang! – rather than any sense of an ongoing interaction which it might be possible to halt at different stages. Walking is a rhythmic activity so the walking analogy conveys a sense of interaction and mutual interdependence without quite the same feel of an inevitable end-point. On the other hand the two legs contribute absolutely equally which may not be quite the impression one wants to give. The tasty sponge cake analogy captures another important aspect of gene-environment interactions. Once the interaction has occurred it cannot be undone, and in the same way once the cake is baked there is no way of recreating the eggs and flour.

Question 1.5

(a) Partly true. In addition the past environment of an individual will have effects on their present phenotype, e.g. phenylketonuria (PKU), thrifty phenotype, etc.

(b) Partly true. However, recombination and independent assortment also lead to individual differences in genotype.

(c) False. *SRY* promotes differentiation of the indifferent gonad into a testis.

(d) False. Nearly all the amino acids are coded by two or more codons.

(e) False. The separation of chromosomes during meiosis may proceed incorrectly, resulting in gametes that have extra or too few chromosomes. Fertilization involving such gametes will produce a zygote with an aneuploidy.

(f) Partly true. Up to 50–70% of miscarried fetuses do have chromosome abnormalities but most are aneuploidies in which chromosome numbers are increased or reduced. Polyploidies are also more frequent than structural alterations (Table 1.1).

Question 2.1

REM sleep is called paradoxical sleep because, in behavioural terms, it looks like deep sleep; a person in REM sleep is relaxed and immobile. Their brain activity, however, resembles that of a person who is wide awake. Also, as REM implies, their eyes are moving about; the sleeper is dreaming.

Question 2.2

Deep sleep is characterized by EEG patterns that show distinct 'slow waves' with a period of 0.5 to 2.0 seconds. People woken from deep sleep are typically poorly coordinated and confused. Deep sleep occurs mostly during the first part of a night's sleep.

Question 2.3

The situation arises because your biological clock, which tells your body when it is time to sleep, is out of phase with your environment, which usually dictates that you sleep at night. Depending on where in America you have come from, you will be 4 to 8 hours out of phase and it will take you 4 to 8 days to get fully back to normal.

Question 2.4

As we get older, the duration of night-time sleep falls, from about 16 hours per day in infants to 5 to 10 hours in adults, and we become more likely to take a nap during the day. The proportion of sleep spent in REM sleep falls from about 50% in infants to 20% in old age.

Question 2.5

The restorative theory proposes that sleep has a short-term effect, allowing the body and the brain to recover from daytime activity. The ecological theory suggests that sleep is an adaptive pattern of behaviour (i.e. it increases lifetime fitness) by keeping animals 'out of harm's way' during certain times of day.

Question 2.6

ASPD is a condition in which a person wants to go to sleep early in the evening and to get up early in the morning. People with ASPD are alert and energetic early in the day and become lethargic in the afternoon.

Question 2.7

Predators eat nutrient-rich food and thus need few meals. They thus have a lot of time when they do not need to eat, and so sleep instead. Herbivores eat nutrient-poor food and have to spend a large proportion of their time feeding. They have little 'spare' time for sleeping. This provides support for the ecological theory for the function of sleep.

Question 3.1

(a) False. Sympathetic activity releases adrenalin and noradrenalin, whereas HPA activity releases cortisol.

(b) True.

(c) False. Stress causes the breakdown of stored fats into fatty acids, so if anything, the reverse should be true.

(d) True.

(e) True.

(f) True.

(g) False. Prolonged stress decreases immunoglobulin levels in the saliva.

Question 3.2

The completed table is shown below.

System	Short-term	Long-term
circulation	increase in heart rate and blood pressure	plaque formation and risk of heart disease
immune system	transient increase in function	suppression of function and increased risk of infectious disease
brain	increase in alertness	loss of hippocampal connections and memory formation and function
reproductive system	reduction in sex hormones	loss of desire or sexual dysfunction

Question 3.3

(a) There are many possibilities. You could measure levels of hormones such as cortisol when people arrived for work, or monitor people's heart rate or adrenalin levels in response to talking about their jobs.

(b) If people were given greater control, for example, of the hours they worked, the order in which they did their tasks, or the way they worked together, their levels of stress would be expected to reduce. By giving employees information about future plans, and including them in company decisions, you could give them a greater sense of predictability. Finally, you could provide sports facilities and other outlets for stress.

Question 3.4

There are many different arguments you might have come up with. Here are some of the main ones.

(a) Scientific

For: The stress response is highly conserved and so likely to be similar across different species. It is possible to perform experimental interventions on non-human animals that would not be possible on humans. Therefore knowledge will advance more quickly using animal experiments than working solely on humans.

Against: Different animals have different physiologies and especially different psychologies, so knowledge from animal models will not always be directly applicable to humans. Humans have a far greater capacity to ruminate and worry about the distant future than other species, so the nature of stress may be quite different.

(b) Ethical

For: Stress-related diseases cause untold and probably avoidable human suffering. If animal experiments are the quickest way to obtain knowledge which will help end such suffering, we have an ethical duty to pursue it.

Against: Stress research almost always involves making the animal suffer. Animals cannot choose to take part in such research, nor do they always benefit from the results.

Question 4.1

(a) True. Both spermatogenesis and oogenesis take place within a background of pulsatile release of GnRH by the hypothalamus. GnRH stimulates secretion of the gonadotropins LH and FSH by the anterior pituitary. The gonadotropins play important roles in controlling spermatogenesis and oogenesis.

(b) False. Both spermatogenesis and oogenesis are cyclic. Spermatogenesis is cyclic in that each stem cell in the seminiferous tubules initiates a sequence of mitotic divisions every 16 days. Spermatogenic cycles are not so complex as the menstrual cycles.

(c) True. Spermatogenesis can proceed throughout a male's lifespan, because there are stem cells in the testes. Mitoses of stem cells and their daughter cells produce spermatocytes, which undergo meiosis producing haploid immature sperm, which undergo maturation. In contrast, baby girls are born with all their oocytes, and there are no stem cells in the ovaries. Once the oocytes in the ovaries have been depleted, further generation of oocytes is not possible.

(d) True. In men, circulating testosterone exerts negative feedback on the pituitary decreasing LH secretion and to a lesser extent FSH secretion. (Inhibin provides the major negative feedback control of FSH secretion in men.) In women, circulating oestrogens exert negative feedback control on LH and FSH secretion. (In the late follicular phase, oestrogen exerts positive feedback control on LH secretion causing a surge in blood LH levels.)

(e) False. The epididymis plays an important role in sperm maturation. As spermatozoa pass through the epididymis they are coated with fructose and glycoproteins and are then capable of swimming. Once sperm have been capacitated in the female tract, they can swim to the fallopian tubes.

(f) Partly true. Fertilization involves fusion of an oocyte and a sperm cell, but it is a lengthy process that includes capacitation, initiating processes that dissolve the zona and so help the sperm to penetrate. Fusion of the oocyte with the sperm head forms a zygote with two pronuclei once the second meiotic division of the oocyte is completed. Within 4–7 hours of fusion, the pronuclear membranes break down and the diploid set of chromosomes moves to the centre of the cell. So now the maternal and paternal chromosomes have come together and the first mitosis occurs, forming a 2-celled embryo.

Question 4.2

- Stem cells located at the base of the seminiferous epithelium divide forming groups of spermatocytes, tucked into much larger Sertoli cells.

- Each spermatocyte undergoes meiosis forming four haploid cells. By this stage the developing spermazoa are still associated with Sertoli cells but are closer to the lumen of the tubule.

- As the developing sperm cells mature, they develop the characteristic head and tail structure of the spermatozoa.

- The spermatozoa pass into the lumen of the seminiferous tubule and pass through the epididymis where they are coated in sugars and glycoprotein secretions.

- The mature sperm move into the vas deferens; at this stage the sperm can swim and are ready for ejaculation.

Question 4.3

(i) Figure 4.21a shows that during the early follicular phase of the menstrual cycle (day 8), levels of LH fluctuate at around 15–20 mU ml^{-1} blood; levels of FSH fluctuate around 10 mU ml^{-1}. In contrast, in the post-menopausal woman, FSH levels fluctuate around 120 mU ml^{-1}, considerably higher than levels of LH which fluctuate between 60 and 80 mU ml^{-1}.

(ii) The ovaries of the post-menopausal woman are not producing any oestrogen or progesterone so there is no negative feedback acting on the anterior pituitary. Therefore FSH and LH are secreted at maximal rates thereby reaching the high levels shown in Figure 4.21b.

Question 4.4

Combined oral contraceptive pills contain oestrogens and progestins. High blood progesterone depresses levels of plasma FSH and LH by negative feedback (Section 4.3.2), suppressing secretion of these hormones by the anterior pituitary. High blood progesterone levels also suppress the positive feedback response of the pituitary to oestrogen, so that there is no LH surge and ovulation is blocked. Normally in the luteal phase of the menstrual cycle, high progesterone suppresses FSH preventing the initiation of growth of primordial follicles and a new menstrual cycle.

Question 4.5

It is possible that a blastocyst may have begun or even completed implantation but then failed for various reasons, including chromosomal abnormality, gene mutation, or failure of the corpus luteum to respond to the hCG.

Question 4.6

Jane, the recipient of the blastocyst, needs to take oestrogen and progesterone for some days prior to embryo transfer. High blood levels of oestrogen and progesterone mimic the luteal phase of the menstrual cycle (Section 4.3.2) and inhibit secretion of FSH and LH by the pituitary. Low blood levels of FSH and LH mean there is no oocyte development in Jane's own ovaries. Oestrogen and progesterone prepare the uterine lining to receive an implanting embryo. High levels of oestrogen would not initiate an oestrogen surge because progesterone inhibits LH secretion by the pituitary. Oestrogen and progesterone treatment would need to continue after embryo transfer as Jane's ovaries would not have a corpus luteum.

Question 4.7

(i) One option is artificial insemination by donor sperm for Maria. A sperm donor of similar appearance to Siegfried would be selected. Another option would be IVF using Siegfried's sperm extracted from the epididymis or testis. Sperm can be injected beneath the zona of oocytes – subzonal insemination using a micropipette. Intracytoplasmic injection, in which a single sperm cell is injected into an oocyte, can also be used.

(ii) Siegfried's genotype should be checked. If he has Klinefelter's syndrome with genotype XXY, he will have no sperm and use of donor sperm is the only option. There is also the possibility that Siegfried may be carrying a copy of the gene mutation that causes cystic fibrosis, which is linked to congenital absence of the vas deferens. If sperm were extracted from the epididymis or testis for ICSI, there is risk of the offspring inheriting a gene for cystic fibrosis, which should be explained to Siegfried and Maria. If ICSI is possible, and Siegfried's genotype was found to include a gene mutation linked to cystic fibrosis, embryos derived from ICSI should be screened by pre-implantation genetic diagnosis before proceeding with embryo transfer.

ACKNOWLEDGEMENTS

Grateful acknowledgement is made to the following sources for permission to reproduce material within this product.

Figures

Figure 1.3: Science Photo Library; *Figure 1.7*: Prentice, A. M. and Jebb, S. A. (2003) Fast foods, energy density and obesity, *Obesity Reviews*, **4**, Copyright © The International Association for the Study of Obesity; *Figure 1.8*: Ozanne, S. E. and Hales, C. N. (2002) Early programming of glucose-insulin metabolism, *Trends in Endocrinology and Metabolism*, Elsevier Science Ltd.; *Figure 1.10*: Wang, G-J. et al. (2001) Brain dopamine and obesity, *The Lancet*, **357**, Elsevier Science Ltd.; *Figure 1.11*: National Center for Chronic Disease Prevention and Health Promotion, Atlanta, USA; *Figure 1.13*: Courtesy of Caroline Pond, The Open University; *Figure 1.15*: Courtesy of Sheila Dunleavy, The Open University; *Figure 1.16*: Passmore, R. and Robson, J. S. (1980) *A Companion to Medical Studies, Volume 2, Pharmacology, Microbiology, General Pathology and Related Subjects*, 2nd edn, Blackwell Sciences Ltd; *Figure 1.17*: Parkes, C. M. (1986) *Bereavement: Studies of Grief in Adult Life*, 1996 edn, Routledge; *Figure 1.18*: Courtesy of Becky Efthimiou, The Open University.

Figure 2.1: CC Studio/Science Photo Library; *Figure 2.2*: Roberts, M., Reiss, M. and Monger, G. (2000) *Advanced Biology*, Nelson, Copyright © Michael Roberts, Michael Reiss and Grace Monger 2000; *Figure 2.4*: From National Institute of Neurological Disorders and Stroke website. Crown copyright material is reproduced under Class Licence Number C01W0000065 with the permission of the Controller of HMSO and the Queen's Printer for Scotland; *Figure 2.5*: Martini, F. (1998) *Fundamentals of Anatomy and Physiology*, 4th edn, p. 506, Upper Saddle River, NJ: Prentice Hall, © Prentice Hall, reprinted with permission; *Figure 2.6*: G. V. T. Matthews, *Bird Navigation*, Cambridge University Press; *Figure 2.7*: Emlen, S. T. in Farnes, D. S. and King, J. R. (eds) *Avian Biology*, Academic Press Inc., 1975; *Figure 2.8*: Zigmond et al. (1999) *Fundamental Neuroscience*, Copyright © 1999 Academic Press; *Figure 2.9*: Jouvet-Mounier, D., Astic, L. and Lacote, D. (1969) Ontogenesis of the states of sleep in rat, cat and guinea pig during the first postnatal month, *Development Psychobiology*, **2**, 216–239; *Figure 2.10*: Mukhametov, L. M. (1984) *Sleep Mechanisms*, Springer-Verlag.

Figure 3.1: Don B. Stevenson/Alamy; *Figure 3.3a*: Susanne Danegger/NHPA; *Figures 3.3b and 3.9*: Science Photo Library; *Figure 3.8*: Cohen et al. (1991) Psychological stress and susceptibility to the common cold, *New England Journal of Medicine*, **325** (9), Aug 1991; *Figure 3.11*: Magarinos et al. (1996) Chronic psychosocial stress causes apical dendritic atrophy of hippocampal CA3 pyramidal neurons in subordinate tree shrews, *Journal of Neuroscience*, **16** (10), May 1996, Copyright © 1996 Society for Neuroscience; *Figure 3.13*: Daniel Heuclin/NHPA.

INDEX

Entries and page numbers in **bold type** refer to key words which are printed in **bold** in the text. Page numbers in italics are for items mainly or wholly in a figure or table.